THE PSYCHOLOGY
OF GENIUS

Founded by C. K. Ogden

The International Library of Psychology

INDIVIDUAL DIFFERENCES
In 21 Volumes

THE PSYCHOLOGY OF MEN
OF GENIUS

ERNST KRETSCHMER

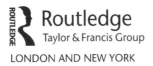

Routledge
Taylor & Francis Group
LONDON AND NEW YORK

First published in 1931 by
Routledge, Trench, Trubner & Co., Ltd.
2 Park Square, Milton Park, Abingdon, Oxfordshire OX14 4RN
711 Third Avenue, New York, NY 10017

First issued in paperback 2014

Routledge is an imprint of the Taylor and Francis Group, an informa business

British Library Cataloguing in Publication Data
A CIP catalogue record for this book
is available from the British Library

The Psychology of Men of Genius
ISBN 0415-21061-5
Individual Differences: 21 Volumes
ISBN 0415-21130-1
The International Library of Psychology: 204 Volumes
ISBN 0415-19132-7

ISBN 13: 978-1-138-88253-9 (pbk)
ISBN 13: 978-0-415-21061-4 (hbk)

CONTENTS

v

CONTENTS

Part Three

PORTRAIT COLLECTION

TRANSLATOR'S FOREWORD

SINCE ancient times, many illuminating observations and many pretentious books have been written about genius, but the real, scientific study of this biological problem began with the modern psychological researches of Dr Lombroso and Sir Francis Galton.

These pioneers started out on two distinct trails which have been followed up—one fitfully, the other systematically—right to the present day. Lombroso pointed to the connection of genius and mental disease, and his paradoxical observations were snatched up and ravelled into a tangle of popular literary discussion and psychoanalytic conjectures. Galton, in his classic *Hereditary Genius*, established the high degree of inheritance of talent among men of genius. His conclusions have been confirmed and expanded by McKeen Cattell's studies of eminent men, and Castle's study of eminent women. They have been developed in many ways by Havelock Ellis. And finally, the attack which Galton began, and which has been characterised by strict empiricism, precise statistical methods and (wherever possible) psychological measurement, has armed itself with the technique of intelligence testing and gone on to new and permanent conquests in the *Genetic Studies of Genius* emanating from Professor Terman's laboratory.

Kretschmer is not blind to these achievements, but he himself is back on the neglected trail of Lombroso—neglected, that is to say, except for a few isolated psychoanalytic incursions by Freud and Adler. The English-American approach has made progress because of the scientific rigour of its methods, but it has done so at the expense of dividing the subject piecemeal, concentrating on one part, and neglecting other aspects, particularly the emotional side. Kretschmer calls once more for the comprehensive view, and himself illuminates the rich complexity of the conative bases of genius. In a region where so much has been built on the shifting sands of speculation, he erects a structure which will be permanent because he has discovered a rock beneath—one of the few established principles in psychiatry. That basis, largely brought to light by his own researches, is the relation between temperament and bodily structure which he set out in his book *Physique and Character*, now well known to English readers. His distinction between schizothyme and cyclothyme temperaments, is one which has been fruitful in many fields, though rarely so much as in its application to the natural history of genius.

It is unfortunate from the point of view of the psychologist, though not, perhaps, of the general reader, that he has omitted to set out fully the raw material of his statistical conclusions and has not set off his results against a control group of normal persons. Again, in supporting his contention that racial cross-breeding is productive of genius to an unusual extent, he argues from a ' distribution of civilisation ' which differs radically from that established by Huntington (*The Character of Races*, p. 230). Intelligence test measurements with various cross-breeds of white and negro races, show that the mixed-blood types fall between the averages for the two races, and in the position determined by a simple arithmetic combination of the averages of the parental types, *i.e.* ' hybridisation ' brings with it no mysterious access of talent.   Kretschmer, however, seeks to prove that the conative disposition at least, is something other than a mere sum of the parental ones—that cross-breeding leads to unusual temperament and character, even if it does not lead to unusual talent.

Kretschmer's treatment is characterised throughout by rare breadth of vision and catholicity of choice, yet there are a few ways in which his standpoint is peculiarly German and therefore of especial value and interest to the reader only familiar with the English literature on the subject. This is, perhaps, most noticeable in the conception of genius which directs his enquiry.   When we find that Kretschmer rules out, at one stroke, all women—by remarking that every woman genius is so because at heart she is a man— we are reminded of Strindberg, who thought of Germany as the last stronghold of masculinism and fled there when-ever the feminist vigour of his wife offended him beyond bounds.   One might also ask, as Leonard Darwin has recently demanded (*Eugenic Reform*, p. 253), why those who write of genius and compile National Biographies, always give such a huge representation to literary and artistic men, and leave out great business organisers, engineers, etc.   Possibly they feel that the latter already have their reward in the salaries that they command.

However, the conception of genius which Kretschmer adopts — ' those who bring to society new and original values '—is quite as broad as that which defines genius as a high intelligence-quotient, though it may give more play to unnecessary individual differences of opinion.

Out of this clash of conceptions there will arise, providing the contestants are willing to plunge into sufficiently laborious and ingenious scientific work to establish their ground, a refinement and further differentiation of the notion of genius which will place the whole subject on a new footing.

The present work makes a good step in that direction. Its general principles clear up obscurities that have long puzzled thoughtful people. And they do more than that, they provide us with rare insight into the characters of individual men of genius, an insight which the most extensive reading of biographies may have failed to give us. For we are shown some, if not all, of the inner workings below the surface which genius turns to the outer world. At every stage in the unfolding of the argument, one is met by fascinating suggestions and one's glance is continually directed along new vistas of enquiry and research. Finally, Kretschmer has a way of proceeding with scientific analysis without impairing the dramatic, human quality of his material. We are reading a scientific volume which is at the same time a story-book.

R. B. CATTELL.

PREFACE

THE essential parts of this book first appeared in the year 1919 and existed until recently only in the form of lectures (given as single discourses to the public) for an audience with considerable psychological training. In the last few years much of it has been rendered more profound and complete in detail.

The views which I have developed here rest upon the careful examination of a very comprehensive primary source of material in the form of artistic works, but more especially of letters, diaries, memoirs and the original reports of contemporaries. An historico-philological treatment of the material, with special, critical demonstrations from literary sources, lies outside the real goals and the possibilities of such a book as this.

Naturally the previous literature of descriptive pathology and the most important specialist works devoted to the problem of genius have been very widely considered. A comprehensive collation of that literature will be found in Lange - Eichbaum's study, *Genie, Irrsinn und Ruhm*, Munich, 1928. In consonance with the original character of the work as a series of lectures, I have indulged in quotation, even in regard to this literature, very sparingly. Those acquainted with the literature will easily recognise in the appropriate chapters, the introduction of biographical and pathological data from the works of Möbius (Goethe), Sadger (C. F. Meyer) and Jentsch (Robert Mayer) : many pieces have been directly quoted from these three well-known pathographies. The above-mentioned work of Lange-Eichbaum, so momentous in its thought and fundamentals, could not be given fuller consideration in the present volume because the text was already finished when the former work was published. However, I have made short references in the introduction to Lange's conception of genius, and I should like to emphasise here the great importance of his work.

For assistance in the building up of the portrait collection, I am much indebted to my faithful colleague of many years, Herrn Klett of Tübingen.

E. KRETSCHMER.

MARBURG.

INTRODUCTION

This book is concerned entirely with the personality of genius, the laws governing its biological origin and the psychology of its inner instinctive structure. The laws which distinguish genius from the mass of men are dealt with equally with those which demonstrate genius as a typical representative of the workings of normal human impulses and forms of personality. And genius has been regarded too, as a series of points in the great, collective flow of historical culture. But questions of the sociology of genius, the origin of verbal concepts, the growth of fame and hero worship, above all, of the theory of value, must remain untouched. Only indirectly, when opportunity occurs, will light be thrown on this aspect. A systematic and exhaustive presentation of the sociology of genius will be found in Lange-Eichbaum's work.

Only a short explanation of our attitude to the concept of genius is required here. Its complicated origin and its varied reference in the historical development of language have been thoroughly studied by Lange-Eichbaum, who finally gives his preference to the sociological conception of genius as a ' bringer of value.'

Since, in spite of some confusion as to precise definition, there is good agreement in practical speech as to the persons whom we shall refer to as ' men of genius ' and only the normal amount of discussion and uncertainty as the less-famous, border-line cases are approached, it is unnecessary to trouble ourselves intensely with the question.

The personalities which form the material of our research have been selected in the first place according to the purely external criterion of fame—that fame which attaches itself to tangible personal creations, literary or scientific works, works of art, inventions, concrete historical documents, etc. The legendary, archaic-mythological sort of fame which still constitutes the core of the mediæval traditions clinging to saints and heroes is, on the other hand, of little or no use for systematic enquiries into the nature of genius. It supplies in most cases no concrete works or individual characteristics ; indeed fundamentally it has no interest for the living personality itself, but only for the massive effects produced in the outer world. Behind these effects, it worships, really, the supernatural, under the symbol of a name or type, and venerates more wholeheartedly the less it is able to detect that these effects emanate from a natural psychological personality.

Opposed to this, we find the modern conception of genius toned strongly to individuality, however much it may oscillate from time to time back to the archaic saint and hero apotheosis. This attitude is a direct product of modern individualism : in it the personality of the bearer of genius, its peculiarities and its worth stand at the focus of interest.

Again, in the field of modern civilisation, we shall exclude from our reckoning, all the much-advertised record performances of virtuosi, actors, novelists of a passing fashion, journalists and sportsmen. In many ways they provide psychological parallels to the real objects of our study, but essentially, they cater only for their day.

Further, we shall leave out all kinds of highly gifted people who spend their time in the intelligent exercise of traditional occupations and professions, as with the majority of those officials, diplomats and generals whose names history preserves. On that account selection is rendered very difficult when we come to deal with the heroes of world history, for world history is actually built up from the interplay of whole nations and multitudes of influential individual figures in the closest thrust and parry.

Instead of the tangible, self-contained creation of the artist, we encounter here, as touchstone for the intrinsic significance of an eminent personality, only the effects in the outer world, and it is difficult to decide how far these arise from a real mental eminence of the person concerned, how far from the momentum of the collective current of affairs, and how far from weaknesses and mistakes in the opposing players.

Thus it will only be possible to consider in this group men of sharply prominent and clearly effective individuality. Especially will it include the few men who, in ways going beyond merely technical victories and diplomatic alliances, have stamped their personalities on the epochs in which they lived—have indeed made epochs which are not to be thought of apart from themselves. Such men are Cæsar, Luther, Napoleon, Frederick the Great, and Bismarck. The minds that come in question here are mostly of quite exceptional power and versatility, and have usually left behind, as a token of their breadth, books and documents which have attained a lofty intellectual and stylistic position in the world of literature, and which reveal at once the great calibre of their personalities.

But the core of every enquiry into genius, will always be composed of men famed for artistic creation or scientific invention, around whom the conception of genius first grew up. A certain preferential treatment of poets and other productive literary men justifies itself not by any superiority on their part in relation to other groups, but by reason of the unique richness of available documents bearing on their personalities. These are of great psychological value because they have generally been produced continuously over a long period of their lives, because they provide a direct and indirect self-portrait of the writer, the style of which is more subjectively bound up with the personality than are the writings of scientists, and more unambiguously significant than the modes of expression of the painter and musician.

Finally, we shall not, in pursuing the enquiry, be over-anxious to bind ourselves to any narrow definition of genius. We shall follow wherever the general sense of our enquiry leads, here and there, and wherever the realm of original but not highly gifted personalities overlaps with that of brilliant but not especially original natures.

The renown of a man of genius is always strongly conditioned in its growth by a combination of social factors. If, however, one takes as one's criterion the relative permanence of the reputation (in a critical, historical atmosphere ; not in mythological circles), it is possible almost completely to winnow away those reputations arising purely from a happy conjunction of social circumstances or from the stupefying effect of a blatant, psychopathic singularity of person. When a personal product outlasts the passing spirit of its time and continues—to use the Hegelian formula—through the fiery test of the next antitheses, to be gathered up into the following cultural synthesis, then its success is generally grounded in the profound laws running through human psychology. But to give an account of those laws would be an undertaking in itself. In any case the typical ' great men ' who are in fashion for a day are merely lucky swimmers caught on a wave of fashionable feeling, or the idols of cliques, and generally disappear from view in the subsequent historical perspectives of art and science unless they happen to be preserved as curios of the style of their time. Conversely, the unfolding of the spirit of real genius can rarely be, in the end, prevented by the unfavourable atmosphere of a period. Long-persisting mistakes, in the form of quite unjustifiable personal fame, are occasionally encountered among questionable geniuses of action, as in the case of Columbus. For the reasons already given, such persons will commonly be found in this group : the lack of any surviving writings or creative work, renders very difficult any estimation of the real quality of the personality. Finally, where the historical traditions are clouded and full of gaps it is quite impossible to form any scientific judgment. This occurs with many great founders of religion whose personalities are a mere texture of legend. Cases of men who have come to fame in the manner of Columbus, where in fact, some ignorant, problematical adventurer by a stroke of good fortune makes a great discovery which, according to the state of human knowledge at the time, would, without his intervention, have been discovered sooner or later, are extreme cases of a one-sided working of a conjunction of sociological factors. And isolated cases of this kind had better be excluded from our array of genius rather than run the risk of doing damage to the whole tradition of this conception. For the traditional idea of genius pays most attention to the quality of personality and is oblivious to sociological circumstances.

We are therefore of the opinion that the growth of lasting fame around any individual, is determined only by inner psychological conditions on both sides—on the side of society and on the recipient of honours. That is to say that both the personality of the genius, and the works which bear its stamp, contain specific properties upon which society reacts positively with strong judgments of value, in a predetermined way. The precision of collective psychological judgment in the recognition of worth was even emphasised, though somewhat reluctantly, by Schopenhauer. Values attained in this way have ultimately nothing arbitrary and artificial in them, nor are they in any sense *a priori* or metaphysical. Much more are they rigorously determined products of the laws of psychology and the biological needs of mankind ; arising either directly from the human constitution as are certain effects of colour and rhythm, or from the approximately parallel conditions obtaining in large groups of people. The judgment that anything is valuable will, even apart from its application to genius, always be called forth by factors which evoke strong positive feelings, a sense of pleasure and the furtherance of vital needs.

Consequently we shall give the name of genius to those men who are able to arouse permanently, and in the highest degree, that positive, scientifically-grounded feeling of worth and value, in a wide group of human beings. But we shall do so only in those cases where the value arises with psychological necessity, out of the special mental structure of the bringer of value, not where a stroke of luck or some coincidence of factors has thrown it into his lap.

This inner psychological value of genius is now seen to be something quite different from that which the traditional worship of great men tended to hold before us. It consists not only in an endowment of great gifts, which are of course indispensable ; but also, and to a greater extent, in a strained, dynamic quality of the spiritual forces. In other connections this quality is customarily evaluated as sublime and tragic, but much more frequently as something socially negative, diseased, ugly or abominable. The value of the man of genius does not lie in his relation to any arbitrarily chosen standards in morals, æsthetics or the orientation of ideals, but solely in the fact that he is the possessor, largely by inheritance, of a special and peculiar intellectual apparatus : an instrument which, in a higher degree than others, is able to create new values in life and happiness, all of which bear the purely personal stamp of his strange and unique individuality. It is in this sense that we are able to understand the conception which regards genius essentially as the producer of new and original things. That definition had better be replaced by the expression : " the producer of personally stamped, special values." For the purely revolutionary, though a large part of genius, is not the whole. Raphael and Bach, for example, are no upsetters of tradition, rather are they the perfecters of a style handed down to them. The essential thing in their genius, is much more the creation and lifting-up from the stream of every-day, professional, traditional practice of a special, purely personal note which is still recognisable to the expert after the lapse of centuries.

Our exclusive task in this research then, is to reveal the natural laws at work in the person of the genius himself and the mechanism of inheritance which produces him. At the same time we shall endeavour to give a living picture, true to nature in all essentials, of creative personalities.

And we believe that the tragic pathos of men of genius can be more profoundly comprehended through such a detached, truthful, scientific presentation, than by the usual, conventional picture with its over-emphasis, its touching-up and its insincere idealisation.

PART ONE
LAWS

A

FIRST CHAPTER

The Inner Voice

SINCE the Italian alienist, Lombroso, first coined that pregnant expression " genius and madness " there has arisen in educated circles a very lively discussion, which, however, has been forced to close with the recognition that modern psychiatry has been responsible for—some might say guilty of—establishing such a connection. There is no denying that the partial connection of genius and mental derangement is to many people so distressing a notion, and subject to such inferences, that they would prefer to forget about it altogether. Yet the assertion that these qualities are totally unrelated is so mistaken that Lombroso was already able to quote remarks, some two thousand years old, out of antiquity, affirming the inner kinship of genius and insanity. Such is the observation of Aristotle on the Syracusan writer who could make splendid poetry as long as he remained in a state of mania, but was quite unable to write a single passage when he returned to sanity. Or take the following passage, also from Aristotle: " Famous poets, artists and statesmen, frequently suffer from melancholia or madness, as did Ajax. In recent times such a disposition occurred in Socrates, Empedocles, Plato and many others, but especially in our poets." Elsewhere, the saying of Seneca is encountered: " Non est magnum ingenium sine mixtura dementiae ". Lombroso brings forward from a later period, a passage from the French philosopher Diderot, who remarks :

3

" I have often thought that these reserved and melancholy men owe their extraordinary, almost godlike acuteness of insight to a temporary disturbance of their whole mechanism. One may notice how it brings them now to sublime and now to insane thoughts. They themselves fancy that some godlike being rises up within them, seeks them out and uses them. How near is genius to madness ! Yet one is locked up and bound with chains whilst to the other we raise monuments."

What do men of genius themselves say to all this ? Strange it is to notice how differently the average man on the one hand and certain men of genius on the other, regard these exceptional, exalted emotional states, these conditions of mental disease. " Ha, how he raves, the unfortunate—and doesn't know against what he is raving," shouted young Goethe, à propos of himself. Nietzsche, in his holy inspiration, rebukes the inert multitude : " Where is the madness with which you should be inoculated ? " But Schopenhauer says briefly and drily : " Genius is nearer to madness than to the average intellect." Whilst thus many men of genius themselves prize madness and insanity as the highest distinction of the exceptional man—the biographer stands with uplifted hands before him and guards him from desecration by the psychiatrist !

I should like to add here, yet one more fine dictum of Socrates, which, of course, like many things that have come down to us through the Platonic dialogues, is capable of being variously interpreted. Socrates said of philosophers : " There are many who carry the thyrsus, but few bacchantes." In this, he would seem to demand ecstatic emotional conditions in great thinkers and enquirers into truth. Just as Socrates himself ascribed the guidance of his subjective life to his ' daemon ', his inner voice, so also, the related idea of daemoniacal possession is found everywhere among ancient peoples and has been carried thence into more recent times in connection with epileptics and the mentally diseased. We find that in primitive folk consciousness, the three circles of ideas connected with good and evil genius, possession by gods and by devils and mental disease, were never clearly separated. Similarly, the half-mythological forerunners of what to-day we should call the naturalist or medical man of genius, for example, the Faust figure and related types of the Middle Ages, were easily transformed in popular imagination to wizards who stood in league with the same devil as entered into a ' possessed ', mentally-diseased person.

If we really wish to get nearer to the problem of mental aberration and genius, we must ask of the facts themselves. We can ascertain in the first place how many men of genius have been in the strict sense of the word insane, or who have later become mentally diseased. Their number is by no means small. I can recall, to mention only a few of the most famous names, the philosophers Rousseau and Nietzsche, the scientists Galton, Newton and Robert Mayer, the old field-marshal Blücher, the poets and writers Tasso, Kleist, Hölderlin, C. F. Meyer, Lenau, Maupassant, Dostoievsky and Strindberg, also Rethel and Van Gogh, and the composers Schumann and Hugo Wolf.

But if now I proceed to enumerate alongside these clear cases of mental disease, all those severely psychopathic personalities of the type of Michelangelo, Byron, Grillparzer and Platen, with all the isolated psychopathic traits, hysterical and paranoiac reactions, and all abnormal forms of sensibility, such as are encountered at every step in the lives of men of genius, I should not come so easily to the end of my list.

Since it is only with difficulty possible to fix the lower limit to the capacities which we describe as belonging to the realm of genius, it is scarcely practicable to aim at percentage figures to show the degree of overlap of genius and the psychopathic disposition. Only this much can one say : that mental disease, and more especially, those ill-defined conditions on the boundary of mental disease, are decidedly more frequent among men of genius, at least in certain groups, than they are among the general population. This is the fact which sets us off on our trail of reasoning.

Why now does one run against such powerful opposition when one reasserts this fact ? And why does this fact only reveal itself when one takes the trouble to study original material, remaining hidden, painted over and touched up in traditional biography ? Largely owing to the prejudice of ' psychopathic inferiority ' ; the opinion that the mentally sound are always superior to the less spiritually normal, not only in a biological, but also in a social, sense. Now, to be completely healthy in mind is very agreeable, but never, in itself, meritorious. The mentally normal man is, according to the conception itself, identical with the typical man, the average man, the philistine. I shall refer later to the scientific conception of normality. For the present, we may say that a sound mind is possessed by the man who is emotionally in a state of stable equilibrium and who has a general feeling of well-being. Peace of mind and restful emotions, however, have never been spurs to great deeds.

To be psychopathic is always a misfortune, but it is a condition which occasionally leads one to great honour. Possibly you have already, at some time, wondered why the man of genius toils through his life as through an endless bramble-bush, why he continues his strivings, misunderstood by his teachers, rejected by his parents, and ridiculed or ignored by his acquaintances. You may have wondered why he is always thrown over by his patrons, why the finest prospects are barred from him again and again by what appears to be secret malice, why his whole life wears itself away in care, rage, bitterness and depression.

Certainly a great deal of the blame lies where it has always been looked for : in the environment, in its complete inability to understand anything that is out of the ordinary, and—consciously or unconsciously—in the simple, down-right envy, which commonplace people feel for the strange personality that is overtopping them.

However, the remaining half of the difficulties which beset the life of genius lies in a different place. The healthy, normal-minded man accommodates himself ; he accommodates himself in the end even to the most difficult situations ; he elbows his way through difficulties, has patience, maintains a cheerful spirit and knows how to take life as it is. With sound instinct he finds his way about in social life among other healthy people. And among men of genius, the relatively healthy ones, though afflicted with nervous troubles, have, as in the cases of Goethe and Schiller perhaps, managed after a time, to acquire this power of adapting themselves to their difficult milieu, even though the ability only comes at the end of a very stormy and conflict-ridden period of youthful development. Any man with an apparently normal mental constitution, however, who continually fails to adjust himself is really no healthy-minded being at all. One can think of such careers as those of Michelangelo or Feuerbach—a constant, abrupt alternation of success and failure, a chain of exasperation, despair, and disappointment, of violent scenes and a staggering out of one conflict into another. Now this is the surest medical test for the irregularly-constructed personality, the psychopathic individual ; that in normal, everyday life he is constantly kicking against the rules and running off the rails. And among men of genius we find a considerable number who are certainly unbalanced according to any reliable token. We find them inclined to delusions of persecution, possessed of tendencies to pathological affect reactions, with pronounced mental disease in the next of kin, and the like.

In short the tragic course of the lives of many geniuses can only be rightly understood when seen from two sides. On the one side, the environment ; the normal man with his naïve dislike and envy of the uncommon quality which thrusts itself so tiresomely before his eyes, and, with his healthy coarseness of fibre, which does not permit him to get easily disturbed. On the other side, the genius, the exceptional psychopathic man, with his over-sensitive nerves, his intense emotional reactions, his restricted powers of adaptability, his moods, his whims, his ill-temper. And this same being not only treats the honest, bourgeois citizen all too frequently in an irritating, inconsiderate, haughty manner, but also upsets the lives and strains the patience of those who genuinely love him, who would like to do good to him and further his success.

When the wife of a famous scientist after his death had an audience with the King of Sweden, she responded to a sympathetic enquiry about the dead man with the remark : " Your Majesty, he was intolerable." If all biographers had the honesty of this woman, there would be many pedestals to genius decorated with that inscription.

One reads, with a slight smile of superiority, of these teachers of youthful genius who predicted for its bearer a place in a lunatic asylum, simply because they saw in him a truant and a ne'er-do-well and were blind to his real greatness of spirit. But these teachers were absolutely right in their direct observations, for a certain strangeness and irregularity of character is already there, and may be seen even in the earliest years, though genius can only develop at a much later period. In youth, both dispositions—that which leads to genius and that which causes the genius to run amok socially—develop as a single stem. That again is a fact most clearly recognised by geniuses themselves. Bismarck, as a student, remarked, " I shall become either the greatest vagabond or the first man in Prussia."

And Gottfried Keller has put forward the same observation in a well-known sonnet in which we are shown the two greatest wasters and rogues of their school class, meeting again as they pass by in the glimmer of a street lamp—the one a poet, the other a ragged criminal and vagabond.

The way in which Duke Charles Eugene of Würtemberg schoolmastered the youthful Schiller was certainly very despotic and unintelligent. But that does not mean that the Duke was not, from the standpoint of his own ideals, quite right, when he sought to educate his pupil to the import-ance of orderliness and moderate living. One can scarcely demand that those who have to live with such characters shall be as wise and clever as the biographers who subse-quently survey the whole life course of the genius. At that phase of his life, Schiller did, in fact, offer to the outsider a real problem character, and the picture admits of so little retouching because Schiller was himself in later life its most unsparing critic. He showed in adolescence an astonishing lack of mental symmetry, such as occurs in many cases of typical psychopathic adolescent development. Thousands of mentally abnormal people show at this age the same gestures of genius, the same loud, shouting, boastful, theatrical pose. Yet from these, there develops no genius, only some neglected, foundered, silted-up existence—a slovenly, ineffective student, a coffee-house poet, a common swindler ; at best, an odd, eccentric person or an emigrant to distant parts who has vanished without trace.

Now, just one glance from the individual into the general. Who, in general, makes revolutions and similar decisive movements in political or intellectual history ? Is it, perhaps, the moderate people, the peaceful, considerate, industrious, comfortable souls who attain happiness in these revolutionary catastrophes and achieve self-expression in them ? Is it the great majority of people of all ranks, the men who, considered from the medical point of view, possess the greatest measure of spiritual health and stability ?

The essence of every kind of health, mental as well as physical, consists in a feeling of comfort and well-being and a state of equilibrium. For that reason the mentally sound man, just because he is of a restful spirit and knows how to accommodate himself judiciously, does not, in any reasonably tolerable situation, break out into poetry, revolution or war. Most of the outstanding movements in intellectual culture and politics are born of men who do not possess that feeling of completeness and well-being ; that is to say, speaking as a psychiatrist, of men mentally abnormal, neurotic, psychopathic and mentally diseased. For the less inner equilibrium a person possesses, the more easily will he lose it altogether under the blows of circumstance. Similarly the less he is endowed with that inner feeling of restful well-being, the more easily will the point be reached when outer circumstances become intolerable : thus he is driven to turning things upside-down, long before the patience of healthy people is exhausted.

Let us observe the extremist, radical political elements which, at the revolutionary turning-points of history, command the political situation from both wings, and, impressing their own nervous energy upon the mind of the inert mass between them, stir into ever fresh commotion the spirits of people more inclined to rest and tranquillity than themselves. Do we not invariably find among these extremists, on the one side fanatics, stormy, morose emotionalists, enthusiasts and prophets ; on the other side cynical, decadent men of letters, the wrecked existences of those who have lived too much, the blasé ones who require some new sensation, the gossips, swindlers, poseurs, murderers and perverts ? It is indeed remarkable, when we run over the natural features of these revolutionary types—they are just the same as those which appear in the peace-time practice of the psycho-therapist. You will find them depicted in the psychiatric text-book in the section which deals with borderline conditions. They are the psychopathic ones, those who live in delicate psychological equilibrium, in the broad transition zone between the healthy and the mentally diseased. And truly this holds as much for the highly gifted as for the small fry in the general rabble. They are in part, the same people as pass daily through the hands of us nerve specialists in times of peace, to whom we give help and advice in their spiritual need, and on whom we provide expert opinion for families, officials and the law. They are the people who are unstable and feel themselves askew, who do not fit into normal life, who are tossed here and drift astray there, and who, under unfavourable circumstances, fall ill with paranoiac delusions, attacks of hysteria or maniacal outbursts.

And if we now turn to the leading geniuses of great revolutions, the picture only alters in one respect ; that we now have before us men of surpassing intelligence. These men are in nowise less psychopathic than the mass of subsidiary, revolutionary types. That is a fact already evident in the stormy drama of the German Reformation, and it becomes clearer still as we pass into the bright bio-graphical illumination of more modern times. Let us glance at the most famous names among the intellectual pioneers and active leaders of the French Revolution : Rousseau, Mirabeau, Robespierre. Robespierre, the son of a father smitten with melancholia, the prototype of the schizoid psychopath and the nervous eccentric. Mirabeau, an adventurer with a problematical past, a dégénéré supérieur with a temperament toned to hypomania. And lastly Rousseau, according to the depth and breadth of his intel-lectual creativeness, by far the greatest genius of the three— the philosopher Rousseau, severely mentally diseased with persecutional insanity.

So we may conclude that psychopaths and the mentally diseased play a most important part in the development of national life, a rôle which might be graphically compared to that of the microbe in other organisms. If the intellectual temperature of a period is normal and the social life sound, then the abnormal ones that wander through the mass of healthy people are powerless and ineffective. But if a sore place appears, if the air is close and tense, if there is anything about, which is decayed or corrupt, then the bacteria become at once virulent and active : they penetrate everywhere and bring the whole mass of healthy people into a condition of inflammation and active putrefaction. Hence it is only a small part of the truth when one says that this or that revolutionary fanatic or prophetic idealist has set alight a revolution. The brilliant enthusiast, the radical fanatic and the prophet are always there, just as the tricksters and criminals are—the air is full of them, but only when the spirit of the times gets overheated are they able to produce wars, revolutions and great rearrangements of thought. The psychopaths are always there, but in cool times of peace we give medical reports on them, and in times of social fever— they are our masters.

Among the connections between psychopaths and men of genius at which we have so far glanced are the following : the frequency of psychotics and psychopaths among geniuses, especially in certain groups, such as poets or revolutionary leaders ; similarities in the life curves of geniuses and ordinary psychopaths, particularly in the period of youthful development ; and, in relation to society, the fermentative effect on world history and intellectual movements which emanate from both groups.

Shall we now draw from all this, the conclusion of Lombroso : genius is madness ? Certainly we shall not. But we shall say : genius is, from a purely biological stand-point, an extreme variant of the human species. Such extreme variants show, over and over again in biology, a diminished stability of structure, a heightened tendency to degeneration and, in inheritance, greater difficulties of pro-pagation than are found in the normal individual of the species. I am thinking at the moment, perhaps, chiefly of human giants and dwarfs with their lowered vitality, or of the hypersensitiveness and liability to disease of highly bred, pedigree horses. Hence we shall not be surprised to find that these extreme variants of the human species, the men of genius, show in their psychological structure an unusual instability, and hypersensitiveness, together with a very considerable liability to psychoses, neuroses and psychopathic complaints. This fact is indeed expressed by our statistics. It is still entirely possible, from the standpoint of a philosophical valuation, to consider the genius as the ideal type of the human species, but it would be in complete opposition to weighty scientific evidence, to attempt to assert, as is very frequently done, that genius expresses the highest degree of soundness and capability in the biological sense. Social and biological values are nowhere so sharply separated as they are here.

The biological inferiority of genius to the normal mind, appears not only in statistics of psychopathic incidence, but also very clearly in the hereditary connections of genius. The fate which hangs over the family of the man of genius is part of the deepest tragedy of these strange personalities. In the constancy of its recurrence, it can almost be regarded as a typical feature. Genius is gradually bred in a single family line or in a group of related families. Such highly bred families of talented people are, as could be proved many times over, one of the most frequent preliminary conditions for the rise of genius. But the genius himself cannot be bred further. One of the strangest biological facts is the rapid way in which the stock of genius disappears, as if by a simple law of nature. Many geniuses have been unmarried or childless ; some have been weak in the sexual impulse, or perverted ; others with strong sexual impulses have shown no wish to perpetuate their kind. And even when progeny have existed, there has seldom been much good to report of them. The marked drop in intellectual brilliance in the first generation can scarcely be conceived as anything but a biological anomaly. On the other hand, we find, especially among the progeny of great rulers and artists, a predominance of very unpleasant psychopaths and decadents, indeed the most stunted and degenerate types. This degeneration in the family of genius often announces itself in the generation to which the genius belongs, or even in the preceding one, and generally in the form of psychopathic and psychotic conditions.

Wholesale family decadence occurs with surprising frequency and severity, precisely among the greatest men of genius : I need only refer to the families of Goethe, Byron, Beethoven, Bach, Michelangelo and Feuerbach. One is tempted to say : genius arises in the hereditary process particularly at that point where a highly-gifted family begins to degenerate. The struggle, continued fruitlessly over decades, which such men as Beethoven and Michelangelo had with degenerative processes in their own families, fills us with the profoundest sorrow and sympathy as we read the story of their lives. When one studies a great deal of biographical material carefully, reading beyond the specious phrases in which the facts are dressed up, he cannot remain in doubt, that there exists between genius and the world of psychopathic degeneration, the closest biological connection. With these remarks, we have not exhausted the biological aspects of genius, but only illuminated the most important of them.

At this point, we are forced straightway to the further question : Is this empirically determined, partial connection of genius and psychopathology merely a superficial, non-essential one, or is it a necessary and inward relation ? Otherwise expressed : Is this tendency to disruption which destiny fastens so closely to genius, a regrettable, but unavoid-able accompaniment of extreme biological variation, or is the psychopathic element an absolutely indispensable com-ponent part in the structure of genius ? In a word : is genius genius in spite of this psychopathic component, or because of it ? Now we can be certain from the hereditary relations, that the psychopathic disposition has nothing directly to do with the high degree of talent. There are highly intelligent and mentally deficient individuals among psychopaths just as there are among the mentally healthy. A psychopathic disposition, as such, is certainly no direct ticket of admission to Parnassus. Conversely, it is equally certain, that there are men of the highest capacity who lack just that hall-mark of genius which betokens originality of spiritual production. From a study of the genealogy of men of genius, we conclude that generally, a certain level of mental capacity is developed independently of any psycho-pathic components. A certain heaping-up of mental power occurs, either by some stroke of chance—a favourable combination of inherited qualities directly out of the common people—or, far more frequently, through a fairly systematic elevation of general mental ability or special talents by way of inbreeding in families and castes. I am thinking par-ticularly at the moment, of the very intensive inbreeding in olden times in the music and handicraft guilds, of which perhaps the Bach family is a classical example ; or, of the long-continued inbreeding of ability in the families of clergy-men and state officials such as occurs in the ancestry of many German poets and scholars, especially Goethe, Hölderlin, Morike, Uhland, and Schelling.

From a survey of a great deal of material, it would appear that a most favourable situation for the growth of genius is created at the point where such old, highly-bred families begin to show symptoms of degeneration. To straightforward talent there must be added, to make genius, this ' daemon ', and it seems that the daemon, the inner voice, is founded in the psychopathic element. For the daemoniacal, which is the essence of genius, embraces the inexplicable, the spiritually creative and original, and the whole gamut of strange passions and uncommon ideas. Compared with other gifted members of the same families or stocks, a great proportion of geniuses have been characterised by a certain loosening of their relations to custom and tradition. This disintegration of instinctive life and established ways of thinking, is a process which, at some favourable point, can lead on to new and astonishing rearrangements of ideas. The loosening of mental structure, the plasticity, the hypersensitiveness to fine distinctions and remote relations, the frequently bizarre play of contrasts in the inmost parts of the personality—all these things, conditioned by the passionate quality of genius, its restless internal production, and its immense intellectual range, are part of the daemoniacal element, which is identical with the psychopathic structures in the personality. Generally, in analysing biographical material, it is impossible to separate the daemonic from the psychopathic elements. Certainly for some types of genius, this inner dissolution of the mental structure is an indispensable prelude. Thereby is attained that interplay of contrasting emotions at the core of the personality, that internal instability and lack of symmetry, which an increased tendency to psychopathic reactions is bound to bring about.

But what intensity and what place must the psychopathic element assume in the mentality of a talented individual, in order to act as a daemonic, inspiring influence ? If one

B

looks first at the severe psychoses, it becomes clear that there are degrees of psychical disturbance which exclude at once any effective mental activity and therewith any work of genius. And yet one may not go so far as to say : every psychosis only confounds the intellect and never, even by exception, promotes genius. We must not let the discussion be biassed by the childish conceit of the healthy, normal man, who, on every occasion, smiles his sense of overweening superiority to the mentally deranged person. Again and again the general discussion has been affected by this naïve judgment.

Whoever has had the opportunity of observing with a sympathetic and understanding eye, a considerable number of acute cases of schizophrenia in the early stages of the affliction, cannot but be astonished at times, at the inconceivable power, richness and cosmic breadth of the experiences that suddenly break upon these individuals, even when they have the most commonplace minds. Such experiences, so quickly to be extinguished, may occasionally lift even the most banal natures right out of themselves. In certain circumstances, abnormal ecstatic conditions of this kind, which are milder and do not lead to complete mental collapse, show a great similarity to the inspired experiences of genius, especially in the religious field. Certainly they are nearer to the experiences of genius than to the ordered course of thought in sane people. This expression of psychological opinion, is sometimes extraordinarily repugnant to healthy-minded persons. For just as men have been unable to conceive God as anything other than a magnified human shape, so the average philistine mentality is unable to think of genius as anything but the vast statue of a philistine. In reality, there are cases, rare, it is true, where a psychotic onset brings out exceptional individual talent previously hidden by quite banal modes of thinking, as Vulcan might hurl to the surface some deep-lying rock.

If it is true that the borderline schizophrenic mentality, especially in its ecstatic heights of feeling, and its strange, irrational combinations of mental furniture, can occasionally produce valuable creations in the realm of religion, art and literature, so also can it be regarded as true, that manic-depressive conditions, in their milder half-developed stages, have some relation to creative production. Here we have mainly to consider the hypomanic symptom complex, in its less intense forms, with its inflamed emotional state and its effervescent production of ideas, which has the nature of a mental firework display. In this connection, I am reminded of the strange periodicity which von Möbius demonstrated to exist in the mental life of Goethe. In its depressive phase it produced regularly an insurmountable staleness of emotion and even ill-temper, accompanied by artistic barrenness, whilst the regularly recurring hypomanic wave of high spirits was the bearer of almost all the works of genius which Goethe produced. And this leads one to think of the psychopatho-logical substrate to the Goethe family, which only betrayed itself in Goethe himself in this mild circular oscillation of feeling, so favourable to his genius, but which came to fuller expression in the severe mental derangement of his sister Cornelia. Similarly, Robert Mayer's creations of genius are founded on manic phase oscillations, but of a more violent kind.

Even in such geniuses as Nietzsche and Hugo Wolf, both of whom fell victims in later life to softening of the brain, we can observe for many years before the final collapse, phases of over-heated, genius-bearing productivity. So here, too, it is not unreasonable to ask whether mild toxic stimulation of the brain, a forerunner and herald of the final decay, might not have produced in highly gifted individuals a passing access of genius.

From all this, we may be permitted to assert that mental disease of every kind, leads in the overwhelming majority of cases merely to a diminution of mental power and to ineffectiveness in the social world ; but that in a few exceptional cases of men with quite special mental constitutions and great talents, it leads to a development of the activities of genius. And this stimulation to productive genius comes in the highest degree only in the initial stages and mild, borderline states of mental disease.

What holds for the insane holds also for psychopathic personalities. The majority of psychopaths are defective and subnormal in their social usefulness. But there are special constellations of inherited disposition occurring in highly-gifted men in which the psychopathic element is not merely obstructive but works instead as an indispensable factor in the personality pattern which we recognise as genius. So we are forced to conclude that were we to remove the psychopathic inheritance, the daemonic unrest and mental tension, from the constitution of the man of genius, nothing but an ordinary, talented person would remain. The more one studies biographies, the more one is driven to the viewpoint that the psychopathic component is not merely a regrettable, non-essential accident of biological structure but an intrinsic and necessary part, an indispensable catalyst perhaps, for every form of genius in the strict sense of the term.

Now, concerning psychopaths among men of genius : we have on the one side complete psychopaths, and on the other—and this perhaps the more important—persons in whom a certain psychopathic element is built into the firm structure of an otherwise healthy personality, like an obscure disturbance in a watch normally keeping good time. Among the completely psychopathic there are great geniuses—I am speaking of such characters as Michelangelo and Byron. These geniuses, in their inability to fit into a normal social environment, in the abrupt, inconsequential zigzag of their life-courses, and in their liability to slight, passing attacks of mental disturbance, compare well with the average psychopathic type depicted in text-books. In these completely abnormal men, the psychopathic endowment has its usual fermentative effect, goading its bearer with tormenting impulses high above the path of average talent ; but at the same time, it has a strongly injurious effect upon them. All too frequently such pathological geniuses fail to attain more than once, the greatest heights of creative production, because the disharmony of their natures tears to pieces the symmetry of their creation, and pierces it through and through with discords. But above all, they fail because of the inconstancy of their emotions and the unsteadiness of their wills. Thereby they are prevented from coping successfully with all the obstacles and attacks that they meet, and so come to ultimate shipwreck or impotence. It is such natures that one is inclined above all to describe as genius, meaning thereby such rare but self-destroying personalities as, for instance, the poets Grabbe or Lenz. Here the daemonic feature of the endowment is certainly not lacking, but the other, the sound half, that the really great and effective genius possesses, obviously is ; and it is that which enables him to round off and mature his creations, and which, above all, enables him to make wide and effective contact with the spiritual life of sound, normal people.

Hence it is precisely with the great men of genius, such as Goethe or Bismarck, that we observe a significant give-and-take of the psychopathic component with the firmly integrated mass of a healthy, total personality. And here, psychopathological traits in the nearest blood relations are very evident—in Bismarck's mother and Goethe's sister. Finer analysis then reveals the psychopathic element in the geniuses themselves. It is seen to consist in an extreme sensibility of the emotional life, in an overflow of emotional stimulation into neuropathic reactions of the vegetative nervous system and in related psychogenic reactions which in some ways verge on the hysterical and hypochondriacal. But here, in natures like those of Bismarck and Goethe, the psychopathic admixture works almost entirely for the promotion of genius, shaping the personality to a richer, more highly conscious and more complex form, making fine contrasts and restless hostile impulses, and everywhere developing the keenest sensibilities. The abrupt inner antitheses and the unstable, nervous over-refinement which the admixture of a psychopathic strain brings with it, becomes tamed by the weight of the sound part of the personality and is yoked as a driving force, as an enriching influence, in the integrated, creative activity of genius.

This much one must not forget : that a considerable part of the ordinary, average man is to be found incorporated in the majority of men of genius. The sane, normal citizen, with his fundamental instinct for order, for comfort, for good eating and drinking ; with his solid feeling for duty and citizenship, for office and dignity, for wife and child, looks out at us as an essential part of genius from such works as

Goethe's " Hermann and Dorothea " or Schiller's " Song of the Bell." Just as the highly respectable citizen is little able to see the psychopathic in the real man of genius, so the wholly psychopathic lesser genius remains blind to all that is normal and healthy in the great one. The high-brow, the decadent writer of the metropolis, the revolutionary hero of a day, smile pityingly at Schiller's " Song of the Bell," as, indeed, the degenerate blue-stockings, bookish psychopaths and pundits of the romanticist circles of Tieck and Schlegel have already done. What they fail to see, is that precisely this large ingredient of the normal citizen, with its contribution of close application, constancy, quiet reserve and fresh natural-ness, lifts the true genius, in all his effects, far above and beyond the noisy and transient attacks of those who are merely brilliant.

SECOND CHAPTER

Instinct and Intellect

It is a prejudice, that has been made respectable by the tradition of centuries, to believe that a profound gap separates the animal nature of man from the highest manifestations of his personality. Anyone who wished fully to understand this tendency would need to gather up the leading threads that weave through the historical development of western civilisation, and to illuminate the typical antitheses, God and Devil, Good and Bad, Nature and Civilisation, which, in their turn, derive from a deep-lying ambivalence of psychological impulse.

Our own path, since we are consciously limiting ourselves to a psychological enquiry, must lie in the opposite direction : towards the appreciation of an ever closer connection between man's instinctive nature and his spirituality. If we will truly and rightly understand the subject, there is no other way. Problems of value and morality are not directly concerned in our research. In so far as they intrude indirectly, here and there, our principal concern will be to ask—if an enquiry promises to be fruitful of anything definite—how far the accepted values are genuine values.

We shall concern ourselves mostly with the complicated transformations of instinctive energy which occur, in the first place, within the sex instinct, then, in related impulses, and lastly, in the great human drives to power and to self-submission.

If I put down a list of about forty eminent men in the field of intellect, mostly chosen from the work of Moll, who with some historical probability were homosexual, or showed homoerotic psychical components, either in themselves or in their nearest blood relations, I discover that the statistical inclination of the series is strongly towards the schizothymic temperament and, contrariwise, very little towards the cyclothymic diathesis. We find in this list of famous men who are partly or wholly homoerotic, numerous cases of schizophrenia, *e.g.* the following sufferers from schizophrenic forms of insanity : Louis II of Bavaria, Christian VII of Denmark, Rudolph II of Habsburg and Heinrich von Kleist. Over and above these, there are a number of persons with extreme schizothyme characteristics, *e.g.* Platen, Michelangelo and Grillparzer. If we arrange the whole group in a psychological series, we hit upon a bipolar distribution in the group, similar to that which normally occurs in the circle of schizophrenic insane people. On the one side are gentle, sensitive, hyperaesthetic temperaments, of the kind represented by Platen ; on the other powerful and imperious natures, cold and detached, varying from the imposing geniuses of leadership like Frederick the Great, to the most degenerate despots. And, thrown in as transition phases between both poles, we find such enormous, torn, pathetic and highly dramatic figures as Michelangelo and Kleist, in whom tenderness of spirit is as marked as the will to power.

Kronfeld has studied the types of personality found among homosexuals in the material of the consulting-room. Here, too, the type most easily recognised is the gentle, aesthetic character, and, according to statistical results, it easily predominates. Kronfeld describes the type as sensitive, unstable, shy, neuropathic, weak in will and with a strong tendency to fixation of emotionally toned experiences. It is a type which can easily be over-refined into a wasted, stimulus-hungry, dégénéré supérieur, generally possessed of strongly defined artistic proclivities. Feminine traits are very common in these persons. But the commanding and despotic homosexual is not represented in Kronfeld's study, for the simple reason that he rarely enters a consulting-room. On the other hand certain types are found among Kronfeld's consulting-room material which are never found among geniuses on account of their negligible social power, *e.g.* infantile, weak-minded types.

While we are unfolding these general constitutional relationships, we can, as favourable opportunities occur, follow up the effects which a homosexual component may have on the higher personality of its owner. In addition to the dangerous social situation created for the individual, there is, unmistakably, in the case of gifted persons, a peculiar positive and valuable drive emanating from the sphere of these abnormal instinctive impulses. Thus we encounter, for example, the subject ' Teaching talent and homosexuality ' already in the circles of Plato and Socrates, as a recognised chapter for discussion. From Socrates to Herbart we meet great men who have made a sublimation of their homoerotic instincts in this direction with socially valuable results. Their instincts have been transformed into a powerful and potent desire to teach the young, a desire suffused with love and passion and borne on the wings of idealistic inspiration. Closely related to this sublimated passion for teaching, is the development of special cults of friendship, which are readily built up in literary circles among personalities with homoerotic components. The circle of friends maintained by the poet Gleim is a good example of this process.   The value of this love is perhaps not very great when it expresses itself in the stylistic gush of exchanged letters and poems, but it is of the first order when it urges such men to a reckless and tireless zeal and idealism in helping others working on the same lines, particularly in assisting youthful talent which has touched their souls to sympathy.   Here, love can do great things, even in its homosexual form.   In the realm of plastic art we find two excellent examples of the results of a homosexual endowment : in the personalities of Michelangelo and Winckelmann.   With Michelangelo, it expresses itself in an untiring creation of masculine beauty, accompanied by a proportional neglect, or even masculine transformation, of feminine subjects.   For Winckelmann it was the essential driving force behind his fine and culturally productive enthusiasm for Greek art, which soon passed beyond that to a reawakening of the ideals of Greek culture in all its forms.

Let us now attend for a moment to the psychologically interesting group of power-seeking and algolagnic [1] impulses. They become effective, as is well known, in the pairs of opposites : command—submit ; torture—be tortured. That they are primarily and exclusively coupled with the sexual instinct is very unlikely, yet the connections are profound and numerous.   We shall speak, in what follows, of sadism and masochism, without implying any standpoint in the discussion as to the sexual connection of these instincts, for it is a question which can scarcely ever be decided with certainty.   Since these impulses, especially in their active form, generally encounter an immense resistance and repres-

[1] I employ this term, after Havelock Ellis, as a useful expression to cover both the impulse to seek pain and to inflict it, *i.e.* both sadism and masochism.   Trlr.

sion from the social order, their sublimations and all the indirect ways in which they penetrate to the highest spiritual expression and activity of genius are tortuous, complicated and paradoxical.

These instincts have a direct and systematically-organised field of operations in the realm of military ideals and activities, where we permit them to abreact in a series of crises which bring catastrophe to whole nations. Although their instinctive character is easily recognisable in the destructive brutality of their end effects, they confidently introduce themselves into our systems of altruistic ideals, disguised as models of heroic sacrifice, for it is in that way alone, that civilised consciousness will tolerate them. The civilised man has so far succeeded as little in dispensing with the satisfaction of the impulses to suffer and inflict pain, as he has in recognising them, and calling them by their straightforward, brutal names. Thus arises the characteristic compromise constructions in ethical terminology and in the shaping of ideals. This sadistic-masochistic leitmotiv runs like a thread of scarlet through the history of civilisation. It plays the leading rôle in war and religion. It is hidden a hundred times over in the notions, ' virtue ' and ' duty '. Because of its part in the honouring and admiration of great men it entangles itself deeply with the problem of genius.

One of the simplest, because the most readily permitted, means of expressing the algolagnic impulses, is, as with plain eroticism, the way of phantasy, of artistic and literary presentation. There is no better evidence for the wide resonance of these urges among all human beings, than the rich variety and wide distribution of phantasies in connection with torture and suffering, as is manifested, for example, in the most successful children's stories (Grimm's *Fairy Tales*,

Max and Moritz, Struwwelpeter. In higher forms of literature
writers with strong algolagnic instincts, have exploited the
effects of the terrifying, the fascinatingly-horrible, and the
diabolical. It applies equally to the prolonged, brooding
murder phantasies of Dostoievsky ; the perverse, contradictory and tortured violence of Kleist's characters, which
unloads itself in destructive thunderstorms of emotion, in
hot-blooded frenzies of suppressed eroticism, in the libidinous
picture of a woman cruelly struggling as an Amazon, and,
less obviously, in the cowed and servile woman in Kätchen
von Heilbronn. Changed into more lovely and more spiritual
forms, the same group of instincts are at work in Chamisso's
sympathetic delineation of the loving woman wearing herself
away in slavish but graceful humility (*Life and the love of
woman*), in the story of the bride grievously mangled by a
lion, in the situation where the almost homoerotically
inclined soldier is forced to shoot his greatest friend. In
Wilhelm Busch the same impulses come to an apparently
very different expression in his endless, amusing phantasies
of vexing and teasing : that part of his complex personality
also comes to clear expression, in his ' Essay of the Heart ',
in the epigram about Brouwer's picture.

The realm of ethics and religion, offers one of the largest
fields in which to observe the psychology of the compulsion
neuroses, the partial origin of which, from perverted instinctive structures, has already been cleared up by Freud
and Stekel. Through the recent work of Strohmayer and
Hoffmann, the recognition of this connection has also been
arrived at outside the narrow field of psychoanalysis.
According to my own observations, it must be regarded as
proved that at least a part of the compulsion neuroses
derives, in a variety of highly complicated and roundabout

ways, from a constitutionally abnormal foundation of instincts, especially of the algolagnic impulses. The obtrusive sexual impulses are repudiated by the total personality and kept down by an overgrowth of taboo-like ritual consisting of defence and sin mechanisms. But the more these moral scruples and self-punishments pass over into self-torment, the more they satisfy the masochistic impulse itself. Thereby a vicious circle arises, which, when the instinctive demands are very intense, defies all therapeutic measures. Even apart from this strongly rooted masochistic circle of cause and effect, there exists occasionally a strong moral-religious preoccupation on the part of the patient, with his own instinctive life, which leads in the end, both for neurotic and healthy natures, to a kind of compulsive, constantly recurring play of phantasy, in which there is a definite craving for self-torment. This sexually-conditioned compulsion, occurring in isolated members of a congregation, can give rise to such a passionate zeal for confession that the sufferer becomes a perfect plague to the Catholic priest.

Some interesting observations in the field of ethics, especially in regard to the psychology of the sense of duty, arise from a survey of the compulsion neuroses. That is true of every grade of mind between the average man and the historical heroes of moral idealism, the great theologians, philosophers, revolutionaries and lawgivers who have been exponents of ruthless moral systems. The man with a healthy instinctive constitution appreciates morality as he does the salt in his soup : it is desirable and necessary, but there is no need to take it in its pure form. " Morality is always taken for granted." But it is otherwise with that portion of humanity which possesses an over-developed sense of duty. They are afflicted with gloomy coldness, or some form of pedantry or anxiety. In these symptoms they show the features which normally accompany a compulsion neurosis. The moral emphasis for them lies always on what one ought to do, or is compelled to do, or on the idea of serving and sacrificing oneself. They do not wish to favour themselves with any rest ; they have no time to be tired ; they sacrifice every pleasure in life, their pauses for recreation and their Sunday idleness ; and they endeavour to demand the same from those around them. There is something tormenting in their sense of duty, which becomes a heavy burden to themselves, their family and those who have to serve under them. This does not spring, as it does with some hypomanic persons, from an overflowing joy in power and productivity, which can find no way of exhausting itself, but apparently from abstract idealism, from an a priori Kantian principle. The sharp opposition of this feeling, in its instinctive origin, to the feeling of common humanity, was expressed by Schiller, when, with an eye to Kant, he wrote the well-known epigram :

"I gladly serve friends, but alas I love to do so.
Thus I brood and worry over my lack of virtue."
"There is but one way out: you must try to hate them,
And then do with loathing what duty begs you to do."

Such a feeling of duty can either be directed sadistically to the tormenting of those around one, or, more masochistically, to torturing oneself. In less severe forms and well compensated combinations, such instinctive components can be instrumental in the performance of real ethical acts of the highest order which have led to the greatest developments of world history. In such a monumental personality as Frederick the Great, who shaped the stern old Prussian conception of duty, these traits of cynical coldness, of moods bearing a desire to torment humanity, even cruelty itself, are in no way lacking : they are, indeed, an essential part of the steely hardness of the organisation he created. In the brutal flogging and execution scenes sanctioned by his father and predecessor in power, Frederick William, this tormenting element is quite naïve, clear and scarcely sublimated at all. For whether the instinctive components indicated are to lead to a distorted psychopathetic caricature, or to acts of moral idealism worthy of the utmost admiration, is indeed, a question of their strength and their admixture with other constitutional elements. The urge to cold-blooded cruelty seldom appears among the great figures of world history more crassly than in founders of virtuous communities. The purest and most abstract moral duty, the highest moral idealism are the leading goals of Calvin and Robespierre. Why do they stare so morosely and gloomily ? Why is the executioner always at their side ? They are the great men, who have raised decapitation to a system ; they have slaughtered hecatombs of men in the prime of life upon the altar of virtue ; and those that remain over, they have banished, or driven and tormented them as in a madhouse— all in the name of Good. Is the good not goodness ? As soon as the good strives to be something more than goodness, and morality more than something that is ' understood ', so sure can we be that it has changed its instinctive basis. Duty—asceticism—torture are upward steps, or rather increasing degrees of frankness of the same pain-seeking instinctive mechanism. As soon as morality passes a certain point—it becomes perversion.

Within the frame of purely intellectual activity, the same sense of pronounced moral duty shapes itself in the same characteristic way, as, *e.g.* with Fichte, the strongest exponent of German philosophical Idealism. He had, in every way, the stuff of Robespierre in him. In his private letters, he appears as a totally inconsiderate grasper of power with Machiavellian tactics. His philosophical system, tending as it did to solipsism, appears as the truest intellectual reflection of his fundamental instinctive structure. Intellect is for him an instrument whereby he may live out his subjective life and reign as a despot, unimpeded and without regard to all obstacles in a more or less imaginary world. He leaves the non-self just enough reality to exist as an unessential slave under the yoke of the self. How characteristic is Fichte's mode of expression : " writings as clear as sunlight . . . an attempt to compel the reader to understand." The emphasis lies on " compel ".

The ascetic ideal of life has here in some ways, clear psychological grounds. We call those people ascetics who find pleasure, not in satisfying, but, on the contrary, in dispensing with normal instinctive needs, indeed, in going against them. It deals with a turning-round or to latinise the expression, a perversion, of the primitive directions of instinct, and a perversion in the most varied fields of instinct. In the sense of elementary biology, many forms of asceticism are to be regarded as perversions, however much they lead, from the ethical standpoint, to lofty performances, and however much the ascetic ideal of life has contributed historically to the higher development of humanity, and therewith given powerful momentum to its biological progress. At this point, one must guard at every turn, against the tendency to amalgamate ethical judgment as to worth, with purely biological study of constitution : there is no overlapping of these categories. That the ascetic perversion of impulse is partly constitutionally determined is evidenced

C

by the fact that many men—I have in mind cases on the boundary of schizophrenia—strive for this ideal of life instinctively, indifferent to all counter influences in the environment, whilst conversely, there are men, generally hypo-manic pyknics, who, brought up in a milieu planned on strictly ascetic lines, never acquire inwardly a taste for asceticism.

Now the ascetic ideal of life is a highly complex matter : overflowing altruistic and, metaphysical sensibilities stand side by side with the crudest tendencies to over-estimation of self. Among the simpler constitutional factors, an obvious under-development of many instinctive structures and a genuine absence of many needs, even to the point of autistic, indolent lack of the simplest sensual urges, make predis-posing conditions. Finally, especially among the extremely caricatured representatives of this life-ideal, a clearly per-verted instinctive structure plays the most important rôle. In the sexual sphere, we find particularly, various algolagnic perversions ; in the realm of the nutritional instinct and other simple bodily needs, we note similar, biologically-conditioned perversions, in the form of unusual desires and queer pleasures and displeasures, such as one otherwise sees in pregnant women or hysterics. Thus, Madame de le Mothe-Guyon, the founder of a religious sect in the time of Louis XIV, was impelled in her youth to eat the vomit of the invalids whom she tended.

Love for the diseased, the sick, the decrepit, the dirty and disgusting ; in fact for self-torment and martyrdom, which arises from this particular instinctive basis, can, where the latter is of low intensity and well compensated, lead to some of the finest social sacrifice : but in stronger admixture it commonly leads to useless ascetic mysticism, which, in spite of its religious clothing, is in no way essentially

different from ordinary masochistic and coprophilic perversions. The most lofty, as well as the most remarkable
features of the lives of the saints are frequently entangled
with this group of instincts, and occasionally, the religious
taste of the time has laid greater emphasis on these
peculiarities of perversion than on the good social work
that has been associated with them. Thus, the cloak of
religious genius, of sainthood, has been bestowed on a great
number of spiritual personalities of the highest significance,
but at the same time it has fallen to some, who, to-day,
would no longer be regarded as objects of religious reverence,
but merely as items of sensational press news, and sometimes
even as assignments for the hospital.

This inmost entanglement of valuable spiritual impulses
and activities of religious organisations with outgrowths of
the same instinctive root which shoots out peculiar arabesques
of perverted impulses is found, moreover, in the Renaissance
period itself, as in the peculiar religious lyric to the hollow
wounds of Christ, of Zinzendorf, a work which had its pre-
decessors in similarly directed efforts of mediaeval mysticism.

The urge to power, and the craving for subjection and
humiliation, achieve religious expression not only in the
classical dual rôle of chastising father confessor and sub-
missive penitent (Conrad of Marburg and Saint Elizabeth),
but they can combine in one and the same person, to give
rise to the religious prophet type, an apparently paradoxical
psychological situation. That situation is well illustrated in
the autobiography of Jung Stillings. There we see blind
grovelling before the inner oracular will of God, which gives
an inner blessing and sanction to go out, as God's chosen
tool, to compel all others to obey that will, to lead and
command them.

Now the sexual instinct appears again in the centre of many ascetic systems as the most important object of attention. Here it is largely a question of sublimation of impulse into the sphere of mystical experience, which in its lesser forms, is simply an imaginative translation of erotic wish phantasies into spirituality, and, in its highest development, a direct transformation of erotic excitement into a glowing experience of a sacred union with the divine, which passes almost without thought beyond the boundaries of self into the cosmic.

The strictest ascetics distinguished their own mystical experiences from this related form, by the fact that they aimed not at the joy of union with God, but at an apparently feelingless state, a pure annihilation of all desires. When the instincts are constitutionally weak, this is easily attained. But, apart from this, we shall regard with the utmost scepticism, the alleged absence of instinctive desires in the ascetic attitude to life. At the very point where the ascetic mood of life attained its historical climax, its typical extreme forms developed a little further and broke out into perverted expression, especially of a masochistic-sadistic kind. Eulenburg speaks very aptly of the fashionable ' sports, in which one enjoyed and satisfied the lust for being whipped,' in mediaeval times. He brings forward edifying examples of ecclesiastical criminal cases in which the sublimation of the lust of pain into purely ascetic exercises had gone astray, and in which the religious penitence of scourging has degenerated into direct, algolagnic sexual acts.

Here we must turn to give attention to the constitutional, instinctive structure of prophets and founders of sects, who again have their interesting analogues among men of genius in more modern times. In order to study their nature at first hand, we will take two highly significant examples of this ancient type from the material of our Tübingen clinic : namely, the case which Gaup reported, of Wagner, the mass murderer with Nietzschean-like ideas of his being a Messiah, and the case, studied by Reiss, of the prophet Häusser. We may add to these, the case, which has recently come in for much discussion, of the so-called Königsberg Sulking Sect, with its spiritual head, Ebel. In all these men, otherwise so different in their teachings and personalities, two things stand out uniformly as the main root of the prophetic consciousness. Firstly, there is a tendency for them to overestimate their personal significance, an ambition for an almost godlike rôle of leader. Secondly, there are certain peculiarities of structure in the sexual instincts which interweave with the overvaluation of the self, and work in the closest reciprocity with that tendency to produce the special mentality which entertains prophetic ideas, indeed prophetic delusional systems. Frequently, the lack of unity in the constitutional instinctive endowment, leads, as with the Headmaster Wagner, to a severe dislocation of the whole personality structure. The perverted instinctive components, which are rejected (in this case, feelings of guilt concerning sodomistic acts), disturb the whole delicate self-regarding mechanism in its most sensitive parts and lead to troublesome overcompensation in the form of a self-regarding sentiment diseased to the point of delusions of greatness. Direct outlets for these rejected tendencies are available in the ritual prescribed for the sect by the founder himself. The partial denial of the sex instinct led with Häusser, to exhibitionistic tendencies which were embodied in ceremonies of sanctity and chastity, which he carried out with the women devotees. There is remarkable similarity here to the ceremonial of the Königsberg Sulkers designed by Ebel at the beginning of the nineteenth century, where exhibitionist acts played an essential part in the sanctification cults. In their ceremonies too, as with most similar sects, there was a good deal of very broad and reckless preaching and talking over sexual matters, which tended to pass without any sharp limits, into actual exhibitionism. There are obvious sadistic-masochistic roots in Ebel's idea of mutual flagellation in a half-clothed condition. One is also very much tempted to conclude, that a sadistic component existed in the notoriously abnormal instinctive life of the Headmaster Wagner, especially when one contemplates the extent to which, years before any overt action resulted, he had satiated his thoughts with phantasies of murder.

Because he was a man on a much greater spiritual scale, Nietzsche, historically the clearest of the geniuses possessing a prophetic nature, offers a picture in which the instinctive structure can be more easily viewed. It would be a fascinating task to demonstrate how the tangle of urges to pain and pleasure, to hate and benevolence, to power and to love, impresses its pattern on all phases of his character, from the crudely erotic, to the highest ethical sublimations, and again, through all planes of his teaching. He perceived this quite clearly himself when he said, " The degree and the kind of a man's sexuality, ranges to the highest peaks of his mind." Concerning the crude instinctive root, we find his view in the well-known aphorism : " You are going to a woman ?   Then do not forget the whip ! ", or in his designation of love as " a painful ardour ". From this point we can well follow the play of feelings which led to his ideal of the superman, to his delight in the ' blond beast's ' love of slaughter and his well-thought-out theories in regard to pity and Christian love. Of the latter he said, referring to its growth out of the ancient Jewish religion, " The new love, the most profound and sublime of all forms of love, grew as a branch upon the tree of hatred and revenge." We are able to understand this monstrous one-sidedness, this immense, though distorted, acuteness of vision, when we bring his fundamental philosophical formula, ' love out of hate ', alongside the instinctive formula, ' sensuous pleasure out of pain '.

And a similar interplay of the self-evaluating tendencies, of insufficiency feelings and compensatory exaggerations of self-importance, together with a changed structure of the sexual instincts, is evident in another great prophetic nature —Rousseau. Here, however, the complication of the separate threads of development renders demonstration difficult. He has, himself, given us a picture of his exhibitionistic and masochistic inclinations, and it has been remarked, not without justice, that his unexampled lack of self-conscious embarrassment in exposing his moral life, stands in the closest connection with his exhibitionistic instinctive mechanisms.

In the prophetic work of Strindberg, woman, feminism as a world problem, and as the object of all attempts at reform, stand right at the centre of his picture. The problem of domination and subjection between the sexes, appealed to the same impulses in his character as were concerned in the chain of violent emotional crises, of alternate erotic subjection and persecutory activity, which ran through his married life. His delusions of being persecuted by his wife have the closest relations to his strivings for the rôle of masochistic martyrdom. This overpowering tendency to regard the relation of the sexes exclusively as a problem of power can develop either upon the basis of a peculiar

instinctive structure, or, from certain experiences of humiliation in childhood : both conditions are present in Strindberg.
With Strindberg, precisely as with Nietzsche and Fichte, the
philosophic structure of ideas which, developed in the
highest activities of the mind, was only a kind of reflection,
an intellectual image, of the instinctive structure lying
beneath.

Of equal psychological importance with the two great
groups of homoerotic and algolagnic instincts, are the finer
quantitative variations of the sexual constitution. Here,
above all, one must consider partial disturbances of adolescent
development and the persistence of partial infantilism and
juvenilism, such as one encounters at every step in the
psychology of hysteria and schizophrenia, but, which also
play a part in the constitutional psychology of the highly
gifted.

Among hysterics and schizophrenics, we find failures of
adolescent development to take the normal course, irregular
order of ripening of adolescent characteristics, and persistence
of adolescent traits into later life, with a corresponding
malformation of the adult personality. We find incomplete
recovery from the early fixation on father and mother, or,
the adolescent protest against the parents, accompanied by
retarded development of the capacity to fall in love.
Hysterical women show most frequently a persistence of
the mental traits of early puberty : a combination of physical
aversion to sex with strained erotic phantasy ; momentary
bursts of emotion ; flapperish excitability ; theatrical pathos
alternating with naïve, pouting childishness ; a liking for
loud, brilliant poses ; a playing with the idea of suicide ; in
short, all that mixture of the droll and the tragic in the
attitude to life which characterises a certain phase of puberty.

From the encounter of this immature instinctive constitution with the problems of adult life, especially in the realm of erotic activities, arises so frequently, all those atavistic instinctive reactions and emotional crises which we group under the term hysteria.

Among schizophrenics, and schizoid psychopaths too, there is a persistence of the stigmata of adolescent behaviour. This is not restricted to the sexual instinct, but exists also in the general personality, as a certain awkwardness and undue restraint in mental expression and psychomotor activities. It shows itself again, in autistic day-dreaming, and in an inclination to those forms of sublimation which lead to broad pathos, to idealism remote from worldly things and to boundless metaphysical questionings.

The first appearance of philosophical, metaphysical, speculative modes of thought is to be regarded, among masculine individuals, as a normal characteristic of adolescence. It has strong and typical resemblances in the realm of mental disease to dementia praecox and the schizophrenic mentality. These characteristics distinguish this short period of life as sharply from the naïvety of childish experience, as from the realistic mentality of the mature man, into which the idealism of adolescence tends to submerge itself. Wherever we find in middle age, the centre of gravity of mental interest, still in the realm of pure speculation, we can consider it as biological juvenilism, as an arrested stage of adolescent development. The connection of this life attitude with abnormality of the sexual constitution is especially illuminated by the attitude of philosophers to marriage. Nietzsche remarked, " A married philosopher belongs to the realm of comedy ". Statistics show that, in fact, the frequency of marriage among philosophers is far below the average, and that even where marriages occurred, they led mostly to unhappiness (Socrates, Bacon, Comte, Wolf, D. F. Strauss and others). The age at which marriage took place is also enlightening in regard to the question of arrested development. In Europe, on an average, only 9 per cent. of marriages take place after forty years of age, whereas among philosophers 40 per cent. married so late in life. A classical type of personality among philosophers, however, is the eccentric old bachelor with a very marked aversion for the female sex, as is exemplified in Kant and Schopenhauer. Kant's serving-man, Lampe, never dared inform his master that he was married. Then, when Lampe married a second time, Kant discovered with indignation that he had for years been attended by a married man-servant.

An adolescent fixation similar to that of philosophic interests is shown in an attachment to lyric poetry, which indeed is obviously fed from the springs of youthful love and the constellation of idealistic, enthusiastic emotions connected with them. Again, the great lyric poets themselves have generally shown a preference for this art form, only in their earlier years, and statistics show a rapid quantitative decline of such productivity as middle age is approached, with the substitution of realistically-toned prose narratives. It is not that the capacity to shape lyric poems, itself disappears in later life : it is only the urge to make continued use of it, which does so. Where a rich and genuine lyrical production is continuously maintained, or, as with Goethe, is made to break out again at isolated periods in later life, it is an indication of profoundly atypical constitutional construction, unless, of course, the outbursts are conditioned by strong erotic experiences in actual life.

The love of idealistic pathos, is, up to a certain degree, a specific trait of adolescence : it does not usually occur before that time, and, with the approach of adulthood, it gives way to a permanently realistic attitude. The persistence of idealistic pathos, of the ' divine fire of youth ', can constitute a property of the highest social value, whilst at the same time, aligning itself biologically with the arrested stages of adolescent development. Thus it is, that we find among the greatest inspirers of pathos, especially the writers of tragic drama, partly a tendency to the psychoses of adolescence, notably schizophrenic breakdown, as with Lenz and Kleist, and partly an abnormal instinctive structure, due to peculiarities of development, as with Michelangelo, Kleist and Grillparzer. Then we encounter a number of great writers in the pathetic vein, in whom, without any gross disturbance of the sexual instinct, there is a failure of sexuality to come to complete expression in the mental field, as with such natures as Corneille and Schiller. The work of the former is known everywhere by its exclusive preference for heroic pathos and its disrespect for the erotic motive in drama. And in Schiller, in later life, the erotic played a very small part compared with what was pathetic and philosophical. It is true, that in his riper dramas, he introduced conventional love themes as subsidiary motives, but it is easy to observe how poorly he achieved in these scenes, the natural tone of love, compared to his usual powers of expression. One can perceive at once, indeed, how precisely these dialogues recall the strained, sweet declamations that a youth thinks of at a time when he still has no inner feeling for the real experience of love. Thus, there exist quite clearly, a group of constitutions in which a persistence of the mental attitude of pathos and ethereal idealism, stands in a reciprocal relationship to slight constitutional arrests of adolescent development. In Schiller there was a second, biologically closely-related, failure of adolescence to run its full course. It came out as the leit motif in all his creations and in the emotional attitude to life which persisted through the whole of his life. It was, in fact, the continuation of his protest reaction against the father. He was unable to get beyond the attitude of resistance to authority, which normally constitutes only a short, transitory phase in the psychology of adolescence. In the course of his life, this protest against the father passed on without a break into an aversion for the Duke Karl Eugen who stepped into the place of his father and consciously played that rôle. Thenceforward, from the "Robbers" to "William Tell," it persisted as the inextinguishable point of ignition for all the poetic phantasies depicting patricide and the killing of tyrants, as the source of all revolutionary gestures, and, finally, in a very spiritual, ethically-sublimated form, as the basis of his idealisation of freedom, which blended in a perfect intellectual unity with the human ideals of his time. Luther was modelled on the same type.

The abnormal instinctive constitution which we call narcissism, and which expresses itself in its cruder forms as a naïve love of self, not infrequently leads with men who have the stuff of poets and great men of action in them, to an heroic idealisation of their own personalities, and this in turn, working upon the growing hero-worship of those around them, develops it to still greater proportions. This reaction is very clearly marked with Goethe. In his early life, it was abreacted in Egmont, who appears as a somewhat feminine type, a woman's hero, allowing himself occasionally to be admired, like a peacock ("Look your fill"). In later life, this trait expressed itself in a refined, tamed and stylistic form, as the mien of a life artist, as the bearing of a scholar and poet of princes, in whom there is not lacking a touch of pride, egoism and gallantry. In this polished, stylish presentation of a complete personality, there was embodied, both youthful narcissism and the need for protection felt by a hypersensitive inner life.

In a subgroup of heroes of action, who are partly related to these dramatists, we find sexual frigidity or even a fixed aversion to erotic matters, as with Tilly and Robespierre. This condition is probably connected, to some extent, with abnormal orientation of the instincts, and partly, also, with that general coldness of temperament which has been a leading factor in the success of so many great men of action. Other abnormal instinctive forms, especially of a homosexual kind, are not infrequently found in the masterful natures of great rulers and in their next of kin. I need remind the reader, only, of the immediate family of Louis XIV, Gustavus Adolphus, Frederick the Great and Maria Theresa. Among most of these, as with Frederick the Great particularly, a general coldness of temperament was also an essential factor. However, such frigid natures are only a section, though a fairly appreciable one, of the men who have achieved great success in practical life.

Finally, there remains an extensive group among men of genius, composed of persons with very weak or mediocre development of the elementary instinctive urges, notably, among the more theoretically inclined scholars. Here, very frequently, there is a complete and general freedom from the demands of desire, even in regard to nutrition and general bodily comforts. In the realm of the sexual instinct, we find erotic indifference, indeed there appear to be many, who, purely out of indifference, remained unmarried. Poor bodily development, as with Kant, may be associated with this weakness : in any case asthenic physiques are very common in these groups.

The brief sketch which we have given in this chapter, of the factors and laws which operate in building up the higher life of the soul, has necessarily been confined to the constitutional dynamics of the instinctive life, owing to the manifold nature of the general influences which play a part. But it would be false to maintain, that these important, instinctive, constitutional factors, offer the only key to the higher intellectual activities, just as it would betoken mental blindness of the worst kind, if one refused, on grounds of preconceived philosophical outlook, to see what is plainly recognised by biologists and scientific philosophers, namely, that the instinctive structure of man—to speak again with Nietzsche—' ranges to the uttermost peaks of his spirit.'

The biological tendency to variation in human constitutional instinctive structure, is no more concerned directly with the measuring rod of moral and philosophical values, than are the variations and mutations of plants and animals. Through the chance play of combination in the inherited qualities, there is turned out in each species, a series of variants—valuable, indifferent and disadvantageous. In the variations of human instinctive endowment, possibilities of the highest spiritual development, of self-sacrifice, asceticism, metaphysical yearning, a lofty sense of duty, and a profound idealism, sometimes lie very close to the sources of most unwholesome variants, of perversions, neuroses and psychoses. But here, as in the rest of biology, the stamp of worth and the selection according to value is provided by the interaction of the environment and the organisms.

THIRD CHAPTER

The Chief Forms underlying Personality Differences

THE thoughtful man can find, in the portraits of men of genius, important documents which reveal their personalities. Not only does this apply to the living expression of countenance, but also to the fixed bodily and facial form. Even in ancient times, the physical form, as ' the impressed shape which develops itself as a living thing ', was considered to have some relation to the spiritual nature of the individual. For it is a correct and widespread belief, that genius is born as such, and that it must perfect itself ' according to the laws which caused it to appear '. In other words, original spiritual excellence of performance is possible, only on the basis of special inherited dispositions, which may be assisted in their development by great efforts and favourable influences of the social environment, but which can never be replaced by them.

The proofs of this are already so familiar to everyone in the normal activities of moderately gifted people which we encounter in everyday life, that a demonstration is superfluous. Assertions contrary to this generalisation, which are occasionally encountered, can only be regarded as dogmatic defences connected with certain philosophies of life.

We have pointed out, that the entirely personal creations which are presented to us in great works of art or the labours of scientists, offer an especially fine opportunity to dig out the very kernel of the personality, its intelligence and character, as it occurs in its primary and original condition, bound to the physical inheritance. For these things enable us to assess the real possibilities of an intellect and to fix the unsurpassable limits to which the spiritual development of a man remains bound, in spite of all strivings and all the outer changes of his life. They enable us to select, from the miscellaneous facts and paradoxical groups of character qualities which we find in biographies, those inmost, constantly-recurring, connections and combinations, which constitute the ground-plan of the personality. Thereby we may successfully proceed from the typical social resultants to the underlying biological causes.

In my book *Physique and Character*, I carried the discussion of these constitutional connections also into the realm of genius. There, I developed not only the relations of certain types of mental production to particular psychopathic conditions and forms of mental disturbance, but also definite correspondences between intellectual endowment and external bodily structure. I do not propose here, to repeat the analyses made in that work, but it will be necessary for me to give an outline of the essential conclusions which have a bearing on, and are an integral part of, the study of genius. Also, I must give the reader untrained in psychiatry some little acquaintance with important conceptions to be employed in later chapters.

To understand what we mean by ' primary personality ' —one of the essential conceptions which we shall use—it is necessary to see the secondary superstructure of personality demolished. A classical example of a psychological system which gives due importance to careful analysis of the secondary overgrowth of personality, is found in the teaching of Adler. We are told that the man who, at heart, feels himself to be weak in his struggle with the world, and who nevertheless strives for power, constructs an outer façade to his personality, a series of character manifestations, which, fundamentally, can only be regarded as fictive lines of development, mainly intended as means of self-assurance in the struggle with life. The majority of finished, complex character qualities which we normally see, with all their associated sociological and ethical values, are really not simple, primary factors of personality, but complicated superstructures produced by the interaction of the environment with the actual core of native dispositions. The old physiognomy, just like the popular physiognomy of to-day, concerned itself greatly, to bring these secondary, finished character qualities directly into relation with physical form and feature. It sought, perhaps, to relate a saintly disposition to this form and a devilish nature to that ; it tried to find bodily correlates for nobility, altruism, meanness, pride, vanity, mistrustfulness or religiosity. This way leads nowhere. But behind the outer façade, lies the actual, primary core of personality, as it was given in the first place, unchanging and immovable, in the inherited disposition. It is clear to every scientifically-thinking and philosophically-trained person, that this foundational core of personality cannot consist of developed and consolidated character qualities, but only of certain elementary dispositions, certain tendencies to reaction. These tendencies to reaction are determined by the type of constitution, which, as a simple, elementary disposition, can alone be correlated with physical characters. Moreover, the successful correlation of mental factors with groups of physical features is itself a proof that we have succeeded in getting down to primary mental dispositions.

D

As examples of these elementary dispositions, we have, in the affective field, an habitual tendency to a predominantly merry or predominantly sad and depressed state of mood, to nervous excitability or coolness and stolidity in regard to mental stimuli. These are things which do, in fact, show a strong correlation with physical characters, as is illustrated by the now generally recognised affinity of the manic depressive symptom-complex and the pyknic bodily type.

The discovery of such simple, primary factors, and the tracing of all complicated differences of personality and talent back to a relatively limited number of such original dispositions, is the ultimate goal of our investigations. And for the attainment of that goal we have at hand, in addition to descriptive statistical methods, the most important tool of all—experimental psychology.

We have already carried out a long series of experimental researches in the psychology of perception and thought. For example, a whole group of varied experiments have been designed with the common purpose of showing the ways in which people analyse, in a very short interval of time, a conglomeration of mixed impressions—lights, colours, forms, letters of the alphabet, etc.—suddenly exposed before them. The ability to split up complex, external impressions, we shall describe as ' cleavage capacity '. It is an elementary factor of constitution, and is, for example, much greater among individuals of leptosomatic bodily build, than in those of pyknic physique, whatever the experimental situation may be. This cleavage capacity is a root characteristic to which we can trace back a whole series of complicated mental properties which are of fundamental significance in differentiating types of personality and ability, both with normal people and those bearing the stamp of genius. Such mental characters are : the inclination to abstract or to concrete thinking ; the tendency to analysis or synthesis in reasoning and perception ; and, in the affective life, the tendency, or the absence thereof, to build up emotionally-toned complexes. When combined with other elementary factors, the cleavage capacity determines whether the attitude to life shall be of the idealistic or the realistic kind.

Similar constitutional differences of elementary disposition are found in regard to sensitiveness to colour and form, a matter of especial significance for the world of art. They occur also, in perseveration processes and in the tendency to persistence in activities of thought and will. In the latter field, they are of the utmost importance for distinguishing types of conative temper, of steadiness of variability, of mental receptiveness and ability to concentrate. They are finally of use in distinguishing the various kinds of successful and exceptional performance among famous men.

The bodily characteristics, which, according to studies of the relative frequency of occurrence, indicate such mental dispositions, do not consist of a number of single signs, each of which contributes a new item of information, but, instead, of typical groups of signs, occurring together to present a definite physical type. Such types frequently come to very clear expression in men of genius, as can be seen from a close study of the portrait collection appended to this book. The types of physique which are to be considered in scanning portraits with the object of determining mental disposition, are : firstly, the pyknic ; a rounded, thickset type of bodily build (after the style of Goethe's mother or Alexander von Humboldt) with soft, broad, well-proportioned facial form. Among men, this physique is associated with tendencies to a strong growth of beard and to early baldness. Secondly, we have the leptosomatic physique (occurring with many great philosophers and dramatists), which is characterised by under-development, small proportions and sharp, lean features, which are sometimes also childlike and undeveloped (Kant and Kleist). Thirdly, we have the athletic form, with its typically bony, muscular physique. It is impossible here to enter into the more detailed features and complications of these three main forms. It is impossible, also, to deal with a number of relatively rare and unimportant types and modified forms which remain over. These are mainly the dysplastic forms which appear to be determined by the chemistry of the endocrine glands and are associated with unusual sexual and mental constitutions, with highly variant forms and with arrests of development.

In their diseased mental conditions, the pyknic types show a tendency to periodic oscillations of spirits (Goethe), to temporary alternations of mood between sadness and joy, without any apparent cause. In middle age and the age of retrospection, they are especially liable to melancholic disturbances of emotion. Diseased conditions of this kind, are generally called circular insanities and neuroses.

The small-built, leptosomatic persons, on the other hand, have their most critical age in adolescence, at the time of maturation of the sex instinct. At this period, the more delicate in health among them are much given to tense enthusiasms, anxious philosophical meditation, difficulties with parents, choice of occupation and general environment, and they frequently break into strenuous bursts of activity, which are characteristically followed by excessive relaxation and neglect. In mental disease, they are prone, especially at this period of life, to schizophrenia (Dementia praecox), which may lead to permanent mental breakdown (Hölderlin). Men of athletic physique, generally run parallel to the leptosomatic type, both in their normal and in their pathological psychology. Experiment also shows them to have the same psychological tendencies, though to a somewhat less pronounced degree. In the field of mental disease, they are well represented among the dementia praecox cases, but still more among epileptics. Finally, the type which comprehends all abnormal physiques (Dysplastics) is found most among dementia praecox and epileptic patients and is very rare among those suffering from circular and melancholic insanities.

Among sound, normal people, the differences of bodily type, express themselves above all in differences of temperament ; that is to say, in differences of emotional constitution and mental sensitiveness. These are differences which, however, overlap considerably with what one usually regards as the native endowment in intelligence. Now, proceeding in the first place from the physical differences, we can distinguish six kinds of temperament, three of which are mainly connected with the pyknic physique, and three with the leptosomatic form. Once again the athletic and dysplastic forms run, in the main, parallel to the leptosomes. The temperament which occurs predominantly with pyknics we call cyclothymic, in consideration of their tendency to periodic oscillations of mood. That which occurs mainly with leptosomatic types we call schizothymic, because of their great capacity for splitting up their conscious field into its elements. In both cases the tendencies show themselves as strongly in experiments with sound mentalities, as in the symptoms of the corresponding pathological types. On the basis of actual research, it appears that 95 per cent. of pyknics are of predominantly cyclothyme temperament, and that 70 per cent. of leptosomes are schizothymes. The moods of the cyclothyme lie between the extremes of hilarity, and sorrowful depression. Hence the cyclothymes can be divided into three further temperaments, according to the section of this scale about which the mood hovers. These three temperaments, we call the hypomanic (very cheerful and lively), the syntonic (realistic, practical and humorous) and the soft-melancholic (sad-relaxed). To all three groups of cyclothymes, interest in the external world, open-hearted sociability and good-nature are common features. In contrast to this the schizothyme temperaments have a common inclination to autism, that is, to keeping themselves to themselves, to shy withdrawal from their fellow-men, and to humourless seriousness. Their range of temperaments is not between gay and melancholy states, but between hypersensitiveness and dull, phlegmatic conditions. From this range, results the threefold division of temperaments : hyperaesthetic, that is, highly strung and with a sensitive inner life ; then the middle position occupied by cool, active men of decision, inclined to consistency in thought and general systematisation ; and finally the anaesthetic temperament expressed in the distorted eccentric, the dull and indolent waster.

Throughout the following chapters, we shall use the designations cyclothyme and schizothyme, to cover the whole field of mental dispositions and temperaments, healthy as well as diseased. The terms cycloid and schizoid we shall reserve for the corresponding borderline conditions, whilst

the expressions, circular and schizophrenic we shall apply
to the corresponding insanities.

TYPES OF CONSTITUTION AMONG THE HIGHLY GIFTED.

	CYCLOTHYMES.	SCHIZOTHYMES.
LITERARY MEN	Realists. Humorists	Romanticists. Writers of extreme pathos. ˙Formalists.
SCIENTISTS .	Empiricists describing things just as they appear	Exact logicians. Systematists. Metaphysicians.
LEADERS .	Tough, pushful men. Happy-spirited organisers. Judicious and understanding mediators	Pure idealists. Despots and fanatics. Cold, calculating men.

FOURTH CHAPTER

The Breeding of Talent

IN the origin of genius, we find a coincidence of great talent with some pathological component of character. The latter appears according to the laws which normally cause psychopathic and innate psychotic tendencies to crop up in the inheritance. Now, the problem of talent in genius is merely part of the general problem of the origin of talent. That inherited dispositions, and not environmental factors, are the essential causes of highly talented performances can be regarded as proven, according to the present position of research. Peters collected the school reports of over 1000 children and compared them with those of their parents and grandparents. The children's reports deviated uniformly in the same direction from the middle case (the general average) as did those of their parents ; so that, on an average, the children of the more highly gifted parents were found among the more highly gifted section of children and, conversely, the offspring of the less gifted parents appeared among the less gifted section of the children. It is true that the deviation of any given child from the mid point was, on an average, only about a third of that of its parents. Between grandparents and grandchildren, however, the agreement was only very slightly less.

Statistics which take well-known and famous men as their subject-matter, lead to results which correspond entirely with these. Woods enquired into the social quality of the relatives of 3500 eminent Americans. Whilst the mathematical probability of any American citizen being closely related to one of these eminent men was only about 1 in 500, the actual statistical frequency of relatedness of these men with each other, corresponded to a probability of 1 in 5. Or, if we wish, for the sake of clearness, to express it more naïvely, we could say : these eminent Americans are related among themselves a hundred times more than they are with the rest of the American nation. Many years ago, Galton investigated the relatives of 1000 of the most famous men in England, with very similar results : on an average 100 illustrious men had 31 eminent fathers, 41 eminent sons, 17 eminent grandparents and 14 eminent grandchildren. Precisely similar proportions are found in German records of the breeding of intelligence. Thus, quite recently, H. W. Rath has demonstrated the close blood kinship of a large number of the Swabian poets and thinkers. He showed that Schelling, Hölderlin, Uhland and Mörike had a common descent from the Burkhardt-Bardili family, and, that from these men again, lines of kinship ran out to Hauff, Kerner, Hegel and Mozart. The descent of Goethe from Lucas Cranach, has been clearly shown in Sommer's fundamental genealogical studies. In the future, similar comprehensive researches into inheritance will undoubtedly reveal a series of such close blood relationships among our famous men. Especially may we expect this, in certain circumscribed stocks and tribes with an extensive production of genius akin to that of Swabia, e.g., Saxony-Thuringia. Among the families of counts, and other noble families, which have studied and kept records of their ancestry for a very long time, many very impressive examples are known. I need only mention the Oranier family, with its accumulation of gifted people interrelated by ties of blood, among whom are many famous French marshals, famous Hohenzollerns and so on. So that one can already safely assert, that in Germany too, relationships among persons famous in the history of intellectual life, are far more frequent than would be expected on simple statistical probability.

As soon as we go into details, we notice not only inheritance relationships as regards general talent in highly gifted people, but also the arrangement together, in certain sharply defined stocks, of various special talents acquired through breeding from lower levels of talent. Naturally, one frequently encounters men of genius who have sprung up at an unsuspected position in the mass of the people, without any preliminary breeding, apparently by chance. This sometimes happens where it is impossible to demonstrate, either marked gifts in the near relatives, or the necessity of such gifts in the occupations which they followed (Kant, Fichte, Hebbel, Haydn and others). It is only to be expected, that such chance, favourable combinations of talent will occasionally occur, according to the laws of probability, among millions of souls. But such occurrences are far from sufficient to satisfy the normal demand for leaders of thought and action in any nation. Rather, must it be acknowledged, that certain families and relatively permanent groups of related individuals, play a larger part than all the rest of the nation in breeding particular forms of talent and genius.

There are, first of all, the families of people engaged in skilled occupations. These play a demonstrably important rôle in the ancestry of great musicians and painters. Firstly, we find that men with the gifts of genius descend from skilled workers or from people assiduously engaged in occupations requiring the same kind of talent as they themselves possess, or they had such people in their next of kin. I can name from among famous musicians in this situation : D'Albert, Beethoven, Boccherini, Brahms, Bruckner, Cherubini, Hummel, Löwe, Lully, Mozart, Offenbach, Rameau, Reger, Schubert, Stamitz, R. Strauss and Vivaldi ; and from among famous painters : Böcklin, Cranach, Dürer, Holbein, Menzel, Piloty, Raphael, L. Richter, Hans Thoma and others. Secondly, in the most extreme cases, there grow up even whole families of people, famous for their great talent, as is true to some extent of the great families of musicians : Bach, Benda, Couperin, Johann Strauss. As bearers of musical inheritance contributing to the rise of genius, we find, in a very high degree, village schoolmasters and choirmasters, then come simple professional musicians (orchestral players, bandmasters, etc.), and finally, talented dilettante. On the other hand, among the next of kin and in the ancestry of great painters, we find a fair number of quite unknown art workers (Böcklin) and even simple workers in arts and crafts, such as lithographers (Menzel, Piloty), copper-plate engravers (L. Richter), goldsmiths (Dürer), or, with H. Thoma, Black Forest clock painters.

A second group of the most conspicuous importance in the breeding of genius in Germany, is comprised by the old families of scholars and clergymen. Again we are faced with a group possessed of talent running sharply in one direction. They have, indeed, produced a few celebrated musicians (Schumann) and painters (Feuerbach). They have also, at times, given birth to political leaders. In modern France (in contrast to Germany) they contribute a considerable number to the ranks of leading politicians. But in Germany they constitute, in a very comprehensive way, the main hereditary soil for the raising of philosophers and men of letters. The two latter classes are found in Germany as part of a unified, almost isolated hereditary group. The same families produce both forms of talent, indeed, both endowments are frequently mixed in the gifts of any single genius : the philosophers are also poets (Schelling, Nietzsche) and the poets are scholars and thinkers (Lessing, Herder, Schiller, Hölderlin, Uhland). This is beautifully apparent in the great groups of Swabian poets and philosophers. The great, no less than the smaller names among them, are derived, with a few exceptions, from the same class of people. And this class is sharply defined, almost in a compartment by itself, according to race, processes of education, social position and, above all, interrelation by blood. Their genealogical lines are en-tangled on all sides ; the same well-known family names crop up again and again in the ancestry of most of these famous men. In other words, these geniuses are only the high lights of talent which catch the eye in a great, century-old family, bred to a uniformly high level from the basis of the general intelligent citizen, a family moreover, which has distinguished itself largely by the high quality of its endow-ment, rather than by any specific direction of talent developed in single members. Even in Schiller's family, which bears the only great name standing outside this old Swabian aristocracy of intelligence, the same type of family develop-ment is soon evident (one cousin was a clergyman, the father was an active writer, and Schiller himself was designed for the ministry). In the Swabian example one can already perceive how a selection, in respect of general gifts, tends to be followed by further breeding, within the chosen group, of a definite direction of talent. Since the need for trained lawyers and doctors was relatively very small in earlier centuries, it happened, that those trained in theology, who also occupied most high official positions, easily predominated, from the point of view of numbers, in the body of the learned professions. That explains their easy numerical predominance in most of the old German families of great intellectual distinction. Admission to theological studies was regulated, even in the school years, by a series of really difficult examinations (as far as the Swabian example is concerned). Thereby, a continuous selection of ability took place, which acted equally upon children who already belonged to that class, and upon those who were newly entering it. And for centuries, this selection was solely on a basis of proficiency in humanistic studies. That could lead to an increasing preponderance, only of abilities of a logical, abstract and linguistic nature. Other abilities, *e.g.* in painting, music or practical politics, might be present in the high level of purely general ability, but there was no special selection going on in their favour. Doubtless similar breeding went on in the old families of lawyers and doctors, but, for the reasons already given, these families play no large part.

Now, the families picked out in this way, by tests of humanistic ability, married very largely into each other and within the territorial boundaries of the small states and principalities in which they lived, as can readily be seen from their genealogical records. If one could survey the whole net of hereditary relationships in the old families of intelligentsia, with accurate knowledge of pedigree and ancestor documents, he would certainly find that the most

famous men of talent in these families, are themselves more
closely related than previous enquiries have yet recognised.
Through these two factors ; the selection of special forms
of ability by examination and the predominance of the
practice of marrying into families in the same position, the
old humanistic-clerical ability was bred to the high level it
attained in genius.   It grew ever richer and stronger in
abilities of this kind, and it is no wonder, that out of this
evolutionary breeding, begun in the sixteenth century, there
should appear in the eighteenth and nineteenth centuries,
a whole series of famous names.   They are the names of
highly-talented men who were the almost exclusive possessors
of this particular unified, sharply-defined stamp of exquisite
linguistic and logical skill.   Thus they entered as poets and
great thinkers, or as mixtures of both, into the cultural
history of Germany.

This example of the scholarly intelligentsia of Swabia is
particularly clear and well known to me by reason of certain
special studies of my own and much personal information.
Very similar conditions of school and family selection in a
literary direction appear to have existed in olden times in
Saxony.   There has been a rich production of genius in
this country, notably of poets and philosophers (Lessing,
Nietzsche) which has been based in the first place on the
pre-existence of a generally gifted stock, and secondly, on
the operation of the factors we have just discussed.   Goethe's
ancestral records likewise, show, in their essential components,
particularly in the ancestry of the maternal grandmother,
Lindtheimer, a very dense accumulation of scholarly families,
confined to certain territories, issuing from Hessen and
Thuringia.

As regards military and political talent, it is well known

that in earlier times, the majority of representatives were recruited from the upper and lower nobility. Exactly the same processes of selection and breeding as those just discussed, are found to repeat themselves in these groups. Only here it is relatively difficult to ascertain the real effect of biological selection and relation, owing to the privileged position of the nobility; so that the objection is always possible, that preponderance of the nobility among famous generals and politicians rests upon the purely external privilege of admission to these professions and not upon any real selection according to ability. To which, one must reply that there was naturally a selection of ability in the first place, when the aristocracy arose, and that these privileges would only be kept for a very short time in the continued absence of any corresponding display of capacity. When the differences in ability between class and class even themselves up, the differences in privilege rapidly follow them, as has been demonstrated again and again in modern times.

In general we may say that wherever we see an accumulated and marked development of talent, there we shall find processes of selection and breeding at work. These proceed within social classes or localities, or both, and concentrate at these positions rich endowments of the talents otherwise sparsely and thinly scattered in the whole population. This holds not only for geniuses but for all kinds of high endowment. The process is evident in developing the general level of commercial capability of the patrician families in the old trade towns, and again in the rise of the valuable and irreplaceable old artificer stocks of local industries who develop a marked family inheritance of psychomotor skills, as is perhaps best shown in the fine mechanical industries, particularly watch-making, in Switzerland and the Black Forest.

Although the breeding of outstanding talents is often, owing to the nature of the professional demands, a breeding of specific, one-sided endowments, it sometimes happens that, alongside the qualities which are desired in the first place, there appear also, isolated by-products of breeding. These qualities, which are frequently valuable in other fields of endeavour, are naturally far less numerous in incidence than the principal, specific capability which gives its character to the group occupation. Thus we notice that the nobility, when it begins, after many centuries, to refine itself intellectually (and, biologically, to become over-ripe), frequently brings forth examples of great poetic or artistic talent (Michelangelo, Titian, Kleist, Chamisso, Hardenberg, Eichendorff).

The talent manifested in special gifts bred according to position, is, by its very nature, a narrow one. Every sharply-circumscribed, special talent gives confidence and a firm grasp of things in its own field, but also a lack of understanding for the things which lie outside. Abilities and habits attached to social or geographical position are always, in some sense, limited, dependent on rigid forms and traditions. The prejudice and impediment of position are their natural obverse. How then is it possible for genius to spring from such breeding? For it is precisely men of genius who are everywhere the destroyers of tradition and the constant opponents of the world of rigid forms. Here an important factor is hybridisation, the crossing of various dissimilar directions of talent. In genius the rôle both of inbreeding and cross-breeding has been clearly recognised, particularly by Reibmayer. In cross-breeding we have a process which is also recognised in the biology of plants and animals, and designated in that field as the ' luxuriation of the hybrid '. The hybrid, we find, grows larger and stronger than the parent stocks. When we examine the problem of genius biologically, we come upon just such processes of cross-breeding. Pure races, inbred for very long periods, are often poor in genius to a very marked degree, though they may show a very high general level of capability, as may be seen in the regions of purest Nordic racial elements in North-West Germany, or in the old Lacedaemonians, with their strict racial exclusiveness. On the other hand we find, that when the same race, through conquest or immigration and intermixture at great seaports, becomes fused with other, equally gifted, races, there arises sometimes and after many centuries, with explosive suddenness, a wealth of genius. That can be seen in ancient Greece or the Florentine Renaissance : first a migration of peoples (immigration of strong, warlike races), then, for centuries, a relative intellectual calm, and, finally, a period of abundant genius. Sommer has attempted to show that the impressive roll of personalities with the gift of genius which could be mustered in Florence was mainly determined by the onset of a stronger intermixture between the Germanic military aristocracy and the indigenous, artistically and commercially gifted, citizens. There is much to be said for this hypothesis. In any case, the theory of pure race, the belief that some single, highly gifted race, as, *e.g.* the Nordic race, is the one bearer of all genius, can only be regarded as standing in direct contradiction to a great deal of historical and geographical statistics.

Moreover, the notion of hybridisation is invoked here, not simply in regard to the crossing of races, but in relation

E

to the intermixture of two different groups of people which have been for a long time to some extent isolated and inbred, and have thus taken on a certain stabilised, exclusive character. Native tribes, geographical groups, social classes and families connected by some emphatic biological peculiarity of occupation, form groups of this kind. We notice too, that mixed peoples lying on the border between two different nations (not races), such as the people of the Netherlands, Saxony and Austria show quite an abundant production of genius. Conversely the production of genius, in Germany at least, is just about inversely related to the degree of purity and firmness of establishment of the population. For example, the harvest of genius is remarkably small in North-West Germany and Hessen. Therefore we can say, that the main lines of Reibmayer's theory, despite the absence of our modern knowledge of European ethnology in his day, remain essentially true.

Statistics on the genealogy of individual geniuses also show that these persons are not to be regarded simply as the end product of pure breeding of talent in an exclusive class or geographical area. Much more frequently they are a hybridisation product of such groups. Examples in which genius appears as a mixed inheritance out of different nations, stocks or classes, or as a descendant of immigrant families or parents, are numerous. One might mention Frederick the Great, grandson of a Guelph mésalliance with a Frenchwoman, Mlle. Eleonore d'Olbreuse ; Goethe with an ancestral record of mixed peoples from Thuringia, Hessen and Frankish-Swabia ; Schopenhauer and Beethoven, from immigrant Lowland families ; Mörike, from an immigrant Brandenburg family ; Chopin, and many others. A tabular survey, which could be easily extended, is to be found in Reibmayr.

The mechanism whereby hybridisation produces genius can be clearly and beautifully seen in almost any of the single great personalities we have studied. In extreme cases the cross-breeding produces just that character of ' germinal hostility ', of ' warring heredities ', the important rôle of which in human biology and pathology has been so rightly and strongly emphasised by Hoffmann. There arises a complicated individual psychology in which two abruptly opposed inheritances provide the main structural components and stand, throughout life, in constant mutual strain. This tension works in the first place as a dynamic affect factor. It also produces the unstable equilibrium, the emotional exuberance, and the restless inner drive which lifts genius high above the peaceful exercise of traditional occupations and forbids it satisfaction with the ordinary pleasures of life. In the realm of intellect, it produces a great breadth of spiritual activity, a versatility and complex richness of talent and a certain formidableness of personality.

This kind of constitution is most clearly evident when a genius springs from two widely differing parental temperaments, from a marriage of contrasting natures, a fact which I have demonstrated elsewhere. Goethe's father, possessed of a dry, pedantic earnestness, and his mother, with her sunny, bubbling nature, are polar opposites ; and it is possible, when one succeeds in analysing the temperamental basis of each of Goethe's character traits, to follow these parental lines through all the activities of his life. To the schizothyme temperament of his father, we can trace the formal, classical bent, the earnest industry of the scholar and collector, and the stiff, reserved manner of the high official. To the hypomanic temperament of his mother, he owed his easy, free, sparkling temperament, his genial emotions and his capacity for warm love. Both trends have to a certain extent fused in his life and works, but they can also be found, in other phases of his life, and other artistic creations, standing side by side, without connection. An equally sharp contrast appears in Bismarck, between the blunt realism and unshakable instinctive urges of his father, the country squire, and the sublime intellectual refinement and scholarly proclivities inherited from the city-bred family of his mother, whence he also derived his restless nervous energy, his irritability and his icy coldness.

Cross-breeding produces inner opposites, emotional strains, plasticity of intellect and unevenness of mood, all of which dispose to genius—and to psychopathic complications. Here the problem of hybridisation flows once more into, and becomes intimately mixed with, the question of ' genius and madness '.

FIFTH CHAPTER

Genius and Race

OUR modern investigators of European race problems are constantly in danger of assigning to European civilisation, or to some particular race which they regard as its bearer, an unparalleled value and importance for humanity. Such investigators—and there are few who really succeed in keeping themselves entirely free from this error—always remind me of the highly educated Chinese gentleman who wondered how it could possibly be, that European women were almost all ugly, whereas Chinese women were very seldom so. The voice of our blood will always intrude in the discussion and make us believe that the creations of men of our own race are invariably the most illuminating and the most important. In the second place, it is easy at the present time to credit the supremacy of western culture to the quality of European races, forgetting thereby that those races which are now the bearers of our civilisation were despised barbarians in earlier millenniums, at a time when flowering Asiatic civilisations were produced by other races. A survey of culture at that period might have given rise to estimates of the Nordic race akin to those which we are now accustomed to make of the Negro. It is our own good right to propagate the ideals and further the interests of our own race in the political sphere. But that has nothing to do with the search for scientific knowledge and truth.

In the book of knowledge, the chapter of racial psychology is still a very lamentable one. Not because the statements of race theorisers as to the particular characters of races were entirely wrong, but because these qualities were so arbitrarily picked out that the final pictures were complete misrepresentations. Almost invariably the works on racial psychology are so written that one has no difficulty in perceiving the way in which the author, with a show of scientific methods, is setting out to glorify his own race, or, at least, his own political tendencies and fanatical idealisms. The political label of these writers is revealed to a casual glance at the race types they depict : it stands out large on every page of their books. The writer hates the Jews and is enthusiastic about aristocrats. When he is a Frenchman, he extols the ideals of his own people under the pseudonym ' Celtic race ' ; or, as a German, he honours the Nordic race. One tries, as with every chauvinistic psychology, to find the finest representatives of one's own race and the most miserable specimens of other races. Then one presents them in strong colours, side by side, sketching only the positive, valuable traits of one people and the negative characters of the other, nimbly evading, at the same time, all contrary evidence. Such treatment appears in the otherwise interesting and informative books of Günther, which, by leaving out the most fundamental statistical facts, present the Nordic race as the only one which is basically creative and aspiring, whilst caricaturing the Alpine race (the chief constituent in the populations of southern Germany, France and Italy) as a mob of dull-witted, narrow-minded, slavish, round-headed, sallow-skinned individuals. Precisely the reverse prejudice is found in the inspired panegyrics of Frenchmen and Italians. For them it is just these Alpine and Mediterranean types, these ' Latin races ', which figure as the lively, temperamental, artistic branch of humanity, the producers of genius and the bearers of civilisation, and for which the Nordic race, meaning thereby the English and Prussians, must serve as a mere foil. In this inverted mirror, the Nordic heroes of Günther suddenly appear as an army of lanky, long-headed, flaxen-haired sheep faces ; stiff English governesses, grotesque Prussian lieutenants and high school teachers as we know them in comic papers ; in short, a group of stiff, brutal pedants, lacking in the characteristics of genius.

This path leads, not to the growth of knowledge, but to the bolstering-up of the prejudices, vanities and hatreds of classes, races and nations, and to entirely premature political experiments in population control. Actually, even the physical characterisation of European races is still in its infancy as a science. It is not even certain whether the skull shape, which is the basis of attempts to trace the development of races in prehistoric times, is always inherited with unchanging constancy of form. It is far more likely, according to recent statistics and experiments, especially the contributions of Boas and Eugen Fischer, that it alters rapidly with change of environment. American investigators even assert that the skull form of immigrant families in that country has altered within a few generations. If we think out this matter to its furthest conclusions we arrive at a conception in which the term ' race ' expresses approximately what in plant biology is designated by ' local variety '. In that case the bodily and mental characteristics of race would not be immutable, firmly-linked hereditary root characters, but would only appear as long as the people concerned remained under approximately the same physicochemical conditions of environment in regard to climate, soil, etc. If some of these environmental factors altered, the signs of race conditioned by them, would also alter. It might happen, for example, that a race which has dwelt for as long as one can remember, in a coastal district, and been characterised by blond hair, tallness and a long skull, would produce, on being transferred to a mountain climate, a short-skulled, blond variant, entirely without the admixture of blood of other races.

Then the whole question of the immutability of the mental qualities of races would once more be reduced to uncertainty. Even if we attempted to establish the mental racial types according to the physical forms at present accepted, it would be necessary, first, to obtain far more comprehensive statistics than are at present available, and to advance considerably the psychological study of mental traits in particular races. Only on the basis of sound facts dare one proceed to judgments of racial value. And the verdicts, drawn with due caution, would certainly not lie entirely in favour of any particular race.

Having once and for all thrown out these observations on the complexity and the scientific backwardness of the study of race, we will proceed to avail ourselves of the simplest and most certain facts in regard to types with which the anthropological text-books commonly supply us. With regard to any detail whatsoever, it is far safer to follow calm, matter-of-fact authorities like Eugen Fischer, than the more numerous popular enthusiasts and pro-pagandists. We shall limit our studies to the European races, since for them alone is there a sufficiency of compre-hensive, accessible material.

The Nordic race has its strongest and relatively purest

distribution in the German north-east coast-lands, in England and in Scandinavia. As one passes towards south Germany, it becomes ever more strongly mixed with the Alpine race. In pursuing this study, we will leave out, owing to the insufficiency of psychological research, the Dinaric race, which runs into south-eastern Germany. Thus the difference between the nature of north and of south Germany is roughly described by saying that south Germany is, on an average, more Alpine and the north more purely Nordic in type. The Nordic race is described by anthropologists as follows. In build, tall and slim, tending rather to leanness and with long limbs. The skull is long and narrow and the occiput projects outwards, well beyond the line of the neck. The face is equally long and narrow, and the nose prominent and slender. The chin springs forward in a clear line ; the cheeks are thin and not at all prominent. The hair is soft and blond, and the skin, which is clear and very light in tint, permits the capillary blood to be seen through it.

The Alpine race, on the other hand, is of middling stature, compact, underset, short-limbed and inclined to corpulency ; the skull is round and short ; the skin (according to the observations of Günther) is somewhat opaque, veiling the blood, sallow and yellowish. The hair and eyes are brown ; the hair thick, straight and stiff but showing a relatively very meagre growth on the chin. Of these physical characteristics, only the hair and eye colour, the skull form and the bodily dimensions have really been established by exact and extensive statistical enquiries : the rest is filled in largely by casual observation and hence should be accepted only with reservations.

Owing to certain obvious resemblances, it has been

suggested that these racial types are identical with the clinical constitution types which recent psychological research has established. The Alpine man is covered by the Pyknic (rotund, underset) type, the Nordic by the leptosomatic (lean, narrowly-built) physique, whilst the Dinaric race is identified with the athletic constitution types. That would be a great boon to racial psychology, for we are well acquainted with the psychological make-up of these constitution types. We know the pyknic man, with his alternation of lively, merry moods and depressed, matter-of-fact outlook, which we describe as a cyclothymic temperament ; equally we understand the leptosome, with his schizothyme nature, his cool exterior and his sensitive, quibbling, withdrawn inner life.

But the question of identity of race and constitution types must be considered to-day as decided, and that in the negative sense. Exact statistical results, such as those of von Rohden, and especially Henckel, tell us that the pyknic and leptosomatic types show no difference in just those characters that are of racial significance : hair and eye colour, skull index and bodily dimensions—the features which at once distinguish the Alpine from the Nordic race. Weidenreich has correctly demonstrated from a quantity of material that broadly- and narrowly-built types occur widely in all nations and all races. Thus the Alpine race is certainly not conterminous with the pyknic, neither is the Nordic race identical with the leptosomatic, constitution type.

However, the possibility remains that among certain races, or mixtures of races, one may produce a greater percentage of pyknic types, another a greater percentage of leptosome variants. In other words, there might not be pyknic and leptosomatic races, but races relatively pyknic or leptosomatic, and correspondingly more cyclothyme or more schizothyme in mentality. There could also be races with a stronger production of athletic physiques, as had been thought of the Dinaric race, but this possibility we will forthwith leave out of our study, for the race is of lesser importance in the psychological, cultural problems of modern Europe. But it is precisely with the two most important races in cultural connections, the Nordic and the Alpine, that the constitution-psychology viewpoint is constantly thrusting itself into prominence, not only in the mutual judgments passed by these peoples, but also in clinical, statistical studies. The frequency of typical circular affective disturbances (which, it will be remembered, have a close relationship to the cyclothymic cast of temperament in normal, healthy people) certainly varies with the racial origin of the group, as also does the incidence of pyknic physiques. I can witness, from my own practice, that there are more affective disturbances of a marked melancholic and manic form in Swabia than in Hessen. From all this, it is clear that racial psychology is not exhausted by the principles of constitutional psychology, but that at best it can be illuminated by them in some of its most important aspects. For race is not resolvable into constitution, nor constitution into race.

When we come to mental endowment, our first resource, in studying the characters of races, lies in the reciprocal judgments and prejudices of peoples, which are embodied in sayings and traditions handed down through the centuries and which naturally contain a kernel of truth (otherwise it would be difficult to explain their psychological origin). We turn to them, however, only because there is an absence

of more exact statistical or experimental data, and we do
so with all caution. On the other hand the specific gifts
of a race or tribe, lend themselves to more certain fixation,
for we have geographical statistics concerning the birth-
places of genius and the distribution of the outstanding
creations and landmarks of civilisation. As soon as one
begins to investigate these statistics with scientific detachment and without factious race prejudice, they speak clearly
and unambiguously. This is particularly true in the discussion as to the partition of talent between the Nordic
and Alpine races, which lie most clearly in the centre of
the more recent developments of civilisation.

If one seeks to examine the relatively Alpine, and also,
perhaps, more pyknic, peoples of south Germany, he will
find, on closer study, that they divide into a more hypomanic
(gay-hot-tempered) section in the Bavarian part and a more
phlegmatic (comfortable-good-natured) variant in Swabia.
It is not without interest that among the south German
peoples, those with the strongest anthropological admixture
of Nordic blood are counted as the most schizothyme in
temperament : the population of Würtemberg shows, on an
average, in addition to its phlegmatic-good-natured side, a
stronger schizoid infusion than the Bavarians on the one
boundary, and the people of Baden on the other. Seen by
the side of the Bavarians, they make a strange contrast,
by reason of their tenacity, their reserve and unbending
stiffness of manner, and their penchant for integrative,
speculative thought.

Conversely, one often notices that the schizothymic,
Nordic visitor from northern Germany, fails to see the
schizothymic element in the Swabian character ; he finds
the local spirit of Swabia emphatically sociable : to him

the cyclothyme side of the south German character is more readily apparent because it offers the most obvious contrast to his own strongly-schizothyme nature.

If we pick up the anthropological map showing German linguistic areas, in which the proportions of Nordic and Alpine elements in the population are also expressed by statistical frequency relations between blonds and brunettes, we find that the population with the greatest percentage of dark-haired people (*i.e.* with 15–20 per cent. of brunettes) is settled in the following territories : the whole of south Germany (including also Austria and Switzerland) from the neighbourhood of the Main to the southern extremities. Strips of dark population stretch out from this area westwards down the Rhine, ending a little below Cologne, and eastwards into Thuringia and Saxony. These zones of dark race intermixture follow almost exactly the areas of those German peoples that are considered to be of ' cheerful disposition ', *i.e.* more cyclothymic in temperament, namely the areas, Rhine-Franconia, Swabia-Alsace, Bavaria-Austria, and the northward extension into Thuringia-Saxony. Within these blocks of strongly Alpine population, two sub-groups can be fairly sharply distinguished. On the one hand stand the Rhenish-Frankish and the Bavarian-Austrian peoples, both of which have a relatively hypomanic dash in their temperamental constitution. That is to say, they are cheerful in thought, sensual, gay, lively and talkative. On the other hand stands the Swabian-Alsatian group, which in Swabia is decidedly phlegmatic, even a little melancholy, and easy-going, and passes towards Alsace into the sunny ' Sommerweste ' and the quiet, easy humour depicted by Mörike, but seldom passes over into lively, hypomanic forms. The dark race area in Switzerland corresponds to the cyclothymic middle position, *i.e.* its people are realistic, capable, fond of festivity, home-loving and industrious. We see, too, in the French character, in addition to the hypomanic foundation, the bourgeois realism which arises from an element of the cyclothymic middle phase : that cyclothymic position perhaps comes to fullest expression in the temperament of the familiar French ' rentier '. We will not enter at this point into a discussion of the schizothyme admixture in these peoples. All of them are, indeed, not purely cyclothymic in temperament, but merely more cyclothymic than the relatively Nordic people of north-west Germany. That the hypomanic component in the gay and lively nature of the south German people is derived from the Alpine racial element, seems a conclusion to which we are ultimately driven by these facts. In the Rhineland and Franconia we have to deal with a mixture of Nordic and Alpine races, but the former can hardly come into question as the bearer of the hypomanic trait. True, the Nordic race is not entirely free from cyclothymic components of temperament (especially in its realism), but in the areas of purest Nordic settlement we find little trace of hypomanic temperaments ; rather do we find the people serious, sadly earnest in their attitude to life, and, in the old epic lays which they produced, positively gloomy.

Moreover, in the settlement areas of the Alpine race which lie outside Germany, namely in France (especially central and south-west), and Italy (mainly upper Italy), we can perceive the same gay, lively strain (the ' Gallic temperament ') which we know to be normally conditioned by the pyknic-cyclothyme component of the Alpine race. Yet we must not overlook, in considering the French and

Italian character, the presence of a very considerable admixture of the Mediterranean race.

The clearest picture of the constitutional temperament contrast between Nordic and Alpine types can best be gained by comparing the people of north-west with those of south-west Germany. In south-east Germany, especially in the Austrian and Bavarian Alps, the Dinaric race is too strongly represented to permit that area to be chosen for purposes of comparison. If one compares the two ' hypomanic ' stocks of Germany—Rhineland-Franconia and Austria-Bavaria—he will find in the latter, especially as it verges on the Alps, a growing element of raw strength, tenacity and stubborn self-will. Since the Nordic race is relatively very weak here, these characters can only be attributed to the infusion of Dinaric blood.

We saw that a spreading wave of cyclothymic temperament areas is splashed out around the Alps, and that its extent is pretty well the same as that of the areas of strongly Alpine population. Where the Alpine population mixes with the Mediterranean race, as in southern France and the southern parts of Italy (which, according to the map of cephalic indexes, must nevertheless contain a considerable Alpine percentage), this cyclothymic admixture assumes in its manifestations, a tone of extremely naïve, childish, carefree sociability and gaiety. It is this group of traits, together with the definitely Mediterranean tendencies to cruelty and wild emotionality, which we are accustomed to speak of as the ' southern temperament '. But in south and middle Germany as far as the Rhineland, and in central France, we find very widespread the same characters, modified a little towards tenacity, seriousness and strength of will by Nordic admixture. Indeed, whichever direction we care to follow outwards from the central Alpine zone, we can perceive that the cyclothyme traits tend to disappear in precise accordance with the diminution of Alpine blood. This is clearly as true in proceeding to more Nordic areas as in moving into Mediterranean zones, and there is every reason to believe that it would hold for the transition to Dinaric regions. Nevertheless, the change is most clearly evident in proceeding to the north, as we have already described.

It must be especially emphasised that the Mediterranean race, on the whole, is far less endowed with the cyclothymic temperament than is the Alpine. There is a widespread tendency to credit the mentality of the Mediterranean race with the Alpine hypomanic traits. The Mediterranean race is physically a small, gracefully-built, medium type. It is softer in outline, especially in the face, than the Nordic type, and the nose is shorter and broader. But compared with the Alpine type the face is narrow and the figure very slim. Illustrations of the Mediterranean type in text-books of anthropology always impress one as handsome, neat and well-proportioned ; they lack the individuality and ' character ' of constitutional physique which is so striking in the Alpine and Nordic races.

It is as futile to study the psychology of the Mediterranean race in the Italians and the southern French, who have an Alpine admixture, as it is to attempt to gather an impression of Nordic psychology from the people of south Germany. Rather should one seek out some region in which the Mediterranean race is relatively pure, such as Spain, or the large Mediterranean islands, e.g. Corsica. Then one can see straight away that these people of the purest Mediterranean regions are much less cyclothymic than those of Italy, southern France, or some parts of south Germany. Distinctly non-cyclothymic and even strong schizothymic traits are evident in these pure Mediterranean peoples. In the history and civilisation of Spain, there are conspicuous examples of serious earnestness, often almost of gloom. We see also, strong tendencies to grandiloquence of style, to all that is aristocratic, solemn and ceremonious. In religion, in place of the joyful appeal to the senses which characterises the Catholicism of the Alpine regions (Italy, southern Germany and France) we find strictness, widely-conceived organisation and masterly consistency (Jesuit order), traits of dark fanaticism (Inquisition) and fervent mysticism. Also in its political relations, this masterful trait is unmistakable ; next to England the greatest colonial expansion among European nations was made by Spain, even though its empire rapidly fell to pieces afterwards. This specific schizothyme group of characters : will to power, religious earnestness, and that significantly contrasting duality of characters—warm mystical feeling with cool detachment in organisation—is possessed by the Spaniard in common with the Nordic race. There are, in addition, tendencies to cruelty and to wild, hasty outbursts of passion, which form the common stigma of all Mediterranean peoples. Yet we must conclude, that there reside in the temperament of the Mediterranean man, certain heightened cyclothymic tendencies, for where the Alpine race mixes with it, as in Italy and the south of France, the Alpine hypomanic tendencies are still more marked, whereas when the Alpine race is blended with Nordic people these tendencies seem to evaporate.

The Dinaric race, the fourth great race of Europe, is lacking in colour, psychologically, compared with the others.

F

This lack of psychological individuality has already been emphasised by E. Fischer in dealing with the closely-related Hither Asiatic race. The Dinaric race has never, either in its pure region of descent, the Balkan mountains, or in the racial mixtures where it predominates, in the eastern Alps, produced an independent culture of high standing or any significant contribution to civilisation. But that does not amount to saying that the race will not do so in the future. Clearly, the gay, lively element in the German-Austrian peoples does not arise from this race, but from the Alpine race, which carries these traits into all its zones of inter-mixture, spread in a wide ring round the Alps. Of the Dinaric race we can only say that it appears but little defined in its mentality and the direction of its energies, apart from its, generally admitted, martial courage and commercial sense. Further it is impossible to go, on account of the dearth of tangible evidence.

It is especially interesting to note how beautifully the specific racial areas and zones of intermixture give their own character to the form of European civilisation within their borders. They break through the apparently even surface of culture and bring to expression the predominant components of temperament in each race. The map of European religions fits closely on the map of racial dis-tribution. Many psychologists have already remarked that Protestantism, with its cool, sober abstraction, its lack of imagery and illustration, and its strong individualism, is usually localised in the areas where the Nordic race is most strongly represented : *i.e.* north Germany, Holland, Scan-dinavia and England. With the south German Alpine stocks there is characteristically a separation into two groups, corresponding to the hypomanic and the phlegmatic varieties. Neglecting minor territorial discrepancies, one can say that the hypomanic Alpine type, in Austria, Bavaria, the Main Valley, the Rhineland and Franconia, has generally remained Catholic ; whilst where the Nordic race has been blended with the more phlegmatic Alpine variant, as in Würtemberg and Switzerland, a second centre of Protestantism has been founded. The most direct, naïve and warm variety of Catholicism, with its direct appeal to the senses, has been most whole-heartedly espoused by the effervescent type of Alpine variant in France and Italy. There we begin to approach the true region of the Mediterranean race, in which, however, a very different variety of Catholicism holds sway. This is the more earnest, fanatical, mystic, strictly-organised Catholicism of Spain, which, with its many schizothyme traits, is sharply distinguished from the cyclothyme Catholicism of the peri-Alpine regions. On the whole, therefore, a fairly precise religious preference according to race can be detected. Protestantism is the religion, firstly, of the predominantly Nordic peoples, and secondly, of the zones where the Nordic race is slightly mixed with the more phlegmatic variant of the Alpine race. Catholicism, however, is the religion of the more hypomanic Alpine areas and the regions of the Mediterranean race.

If we pick out on the map of Europe the birth-places of the greatest geniuses in art and science, and the regions where our most important cultural assets have arisen (*e.g.* architectural inventions), and then superpose this 'map of civilisation' on a map of racial distribution, it becomes strikingly clear that the zones of Nordic-Alpine intermixture have been of quite disproportionately great importance in the more recent development of European culture. The whole zone of Nordic-Alpine intermixture, *i.e.* the area in which both races are present in the population in fairly equal proportions, includes the greater part of France, Holland, Flanders, the greater part of Germany (especially the middle and southern kingdoms of German speech, including the Rhineland, Thuringia and Saxony) and finally, upper and middle Italy. These racial areas are the accepted areas of greatest fertility in regard to the development of European civilisation since the Middle Ages. Around this Nordic-Alpine central zone, lies a circle of peoples with many significant, but much less numerous, contributions to civilisation. This outer ring consists of areas of relatively pure races, namely, that of the Nordic race in Scandinavia, the northern strip of Germany and England ; also that of the Mediterranean race in Spain, the Mediterranean islands, the southern districts of Italy and southern France. Equally worthy of remark, though as yet little productive of genius, is the area of Nordic-Mongolian intermixture in the north-east Slav regions, Russia and Poland. On the other hand the Dinaric-Mongolian intermixture areas in the Balkans have been astonishingly dead, in any cultural sense. Only where the Dinaric race flows over into the Nordic-Alpine zones of fusion, as in Austria, do we find any blooming of civilisation. Naturally all this holds only for the present distribution of civilisation and does not justify us in arguing to the future. In this pretty clear and comprehensive picture of the racial distribution of civilisation in Europe, there is only one questionable point ; that is, in southern England, the chief bearer of English culture. Even that area, however, shows itself on the map as being of distinctly mixed racial composition ; though as yet it is not entirely clear what racial elements are involved. It is fairly certain that there has been some fusion with the Mediterranean race. Günther accepts the contention that, in addition, there has been a slight Alpine admixture. In many ways the mixed racial zone of southern England has marked cultural relationship with the northern parts of the Nordic-Alpine intermixture belt and can be considered along with them.

In any case, one thing is certain ; the highest developments of civilisation have so far arisen in those realms of the Nordic race in which it has become mixed with other, equally gifted, races. This is as true for the modern Nordic-Alpine civilisation as it was for ancient Greece and India. But of these mixtures, that with the Alpine race has perhaps been the most successful, and has led to the most varied, rich and extensive forms of civilisation that have ever existed. Nevertheless, it cannot be denied that the purest areas of Nordic settlement, such as lower Saxony and Frisia in Germany, have shown great richness of character and talent though they have been poor in genius and cultural productions. These facts were already intuitively perceived and statistically demonstrated by Reibmayr, without any inkling of our present information in regard to race and race differences. There can be no doubt that the highest culture up to the present time has had its centre never in Scandinavia, Scotland and the German coast-lands, but always in the zones of racial intermixture. And the slow northward advance of culture in Germany since the eighteenth century has proceeded parallel to the ' de-nordisation ' of that part, *i.e.* the relative increase and infiltration of Alpine blood into north Germany. This says nothing derogatory to the value of the Nordic race, which is clearly written in history, but it speaks against the ideal of pure race, against a one-sided worship of the Nordic peoples and against deprecatory caricatures of other European races.

In the Alpine-Nordic belt of intermingling to which we are referring, practically the whole blossoming of Gothic art ran its course. It saw, too, the birth of the Renaissance-Baroque culture, the classical French civilisation of Louis XIV, the French Enlightenment and the era of Goethe and Beethoven. But it is possible to distinguish within the whole zone, two sub-regions, overlapping at their edges. One is a more northerly and Nordic belt, in which Gothic found its finest expression ; the other, more southerly and Alpine area, was the home of the Renaissance-Baroque culture. According to the temperamental differences corresponding to the differing racial proportions, the first and outer belt is a cool, schizothyme zone ; the second, inner part, an area inhabited by warm, more cyclothyme temperaments.

Gothic seemed to choose as its birth-place, and region of highest fruition, the northern and eastern parts of France (Normandy to Burgundy). Thence it spread most vigorously along the related strips on the racial map which run through north-central France, Flanders, middle and south Germany. In the more strongly Alpine upper Italy, it scarcely gained a footing, whilst south-western France, an Alpine-Mediter-ranean zone of admixture, reacted very weakly to its influence. In the still more Nordic regions (England, northern Germany, Scandinavia), it had noteworthy developments, which, how-ever, were really weak and tardy compared with those just considered. The whole of eastern Europe very quickly lost the Gothic spirit. Now, compared with Renaissance art, the spirit of Gothic is much more schizothyme : rigorous, deeply earnest, metaphysical and ascetic. Its buildings show that contrast of mystic feeling and coolly calculated

design which is so significant and characteristic of schizothyme psychology.

Renaissance-Baroque civilisation flowered, again with
clear racial affinities, in a belt parallel to that of Gothic
and overlapping it in the middle, but distinctly shifted
towards the south. This strip of racial mingling includes
upper and middle Italy, and may even be said to have
its centre of gravity there, that is, in a strongly Alpine
region. France, south and middle Germany, shared that
culture, but the northern lands showed far less real love
for it than they had shown for Gothic. England and
Scandinavia, especially, remained astonishingly quiescent
in this period of art, at least as far as the plastic arts were
concerned.

The realistic, joyful mood of the Renaissance, with its
entirely worldly, earth-loving, pleasure-seeking, constructive,
artistic nature, had, in comparison with the Gothic spirit,
a more cyclothymic infusion, and for that reason it is,
according to the geographical distribution of race, a phenomenon of the Alpine areas. It may be true that a number
of isolated Nordic individuals, even with such marked
schizothymic traits as Michelangelo, appear to lead the
period with their masterly performances, but it must be
remembered that they lived in a flood of life, the mood of
which was entirely different from that of Gothic regions.
So the Renaissance-Baroque spread its monuments most
thickly over the more Alpine parts of the areas of intermixture, *i.e.* in Italy, France, south and central Germany.
The specific mood and spirit of the Renaissance found its
most favourable soil in the great city republics of upper
Italy and southern Germany : Florence, Venice, Nürnberg,
Augsburg, which overflowed with luxury, power, revelry

and artistic culture, and surrounded the Alps like a blossoming garland.

So far, we have intentionally refrained from emphasising the part played by the Nordic population elements in Italy during the Renaissance civilisation. That part has already been amplified sufficiently by other writers. Frequently, with biassed intentions, it has been acclaimed the most important single factor in the rise of Renaissance culture. True, the leading type of the Renaissance is the nearest blood relative of the Scottish noble, Macbeth, or the heroes of the *Nibelungenlied*. Ruthless, individualistic lust for power, the murder of princes, family strife, fratricide, and a bloody rending of their own flesh and blood among the noblest families—this is the story of the Nordic nobility. The ' Blond beast '—that is one face of the Nordic type, from Scotland to Italy. Its other face, expressing the sensitive, metaphysical, idealistic spirit, carried forward the more northerly Gothic atmosphere from the early Renaissance until far into the mature years of that period. It is not these Nordic activities which distinguish so sharply the spirit of the Renaissance from the Gothic culture, but rather those others of which we have spoken. With the rise of the Renaissance movement, and still more completely with its passage into the Baroque period, there came a revolution in the ideal of physical beauty. The fragile, delicate, narrow figures of Gothic and early Renaissance art began to take on a rounded form ; and painters (Palma, Vecchio, Rubens) finally came to revel as much in robust corpulency as they had previously done in slim, stylistic transparency of flesh. The more schizothyme the mood of the time might be, the more did it incline to an asthenic ideal of bodily beauty. The more cyclothyme it became, the more that ideal moved towards the pyknic physique. If this change in artistic and general mood in the life of the times were an act of the Nordic race, it is difficult to see why the artistic epoch found such a small echo in the more purely Nordic nations. We find the view of Sommer much more plausible—that the amazing burst of genius in the Italian Renaissance is traceable to a mixture of bloods, which had been taking place in the preceding period, between the Germanic military aristocracy and the more successful city families risen from the artistically-gifted, native population. This process is very clearly demonstrable in Florence. We have, in fact, simply another example of Alpine-Nordic crossing. From portraits, and the general information regarding the individual geniuses of the Renaissance which has been handed down to us, it does seem likely that the Nordic population provided a good part of the organising energy and leadership which maintained and made possible the intellectual movement. But this Nordic population must already have been enriched considerably by Alpine blood, otherwise it is quite impossible to explain the wholesale outbreak of talent in music and painting during the Renaissance-Baroque period, for it is precisely in these gifts that the purely Nordic areas are weak and the Alpine intermixture zones outstandingly eminent. And it is against all anthropological experience, to suppose that the two races of northern and upper Italy, after living side by side for centuries, should still be found pure in type at the time of the Renaissance.

We see then, quite clearly, that this new European growth of civilisation was determined in its development, not by any community of language, nor by any conditions of commerce and traffic, but mainly by the nature of the racial zones.

The further development of civilisation in Europe is also bound up in the first degree with that part of Europe where the Nordic and Alpine races blend. From the Middle Ages the zone of highest cultural fruition has slowly broadened itself towards the north, without any obvious relation to nationality, as a band stretching roughly from west to east and delimiting the zone of purest Nordic population. It touched England early, which forthwith began to blossom, in the Middle Ages, and is still, to-day, stepping ever more powerfully to the fore. Then it met the German North, the Baltic provinces and Scandinavia, which now go hand in hand with the older regions of culture and show increasing intellectual brilliance, as can be seen from statistics on the birth-places of genius. This cultural development can well be regarded as another aspect of the biological process of ' de-nordisation ' which is apparently going on in Europe. ' De-nordisation ' can be regarded as a slow northward extension of the line at which the Nordic race blends with other, usually Alpine, races. This northward extension of the Nordic-Alpine intermixture zone, which is completing itself before our eyes, can be a matter for congratulation, from the standpoint of civilisation, only in so far as it signifies the hybridisation of equally gifted races, both of which are maintaining their original strength.

Beside this northward extension of the Nordic-Alpine zone of highly-developed civilisation, we encounter, in recent years, the first fruits of the Nordic-Mongolian hybridisation in Russia. As that civilisation is still in its very beginnings, it is impossible to estimate the limits of its ultimate intellectual advance.

In recent European cultural developments it is possible to distinguish once more, the two zones in the Nordic-

Alpine intermixture belt, namely, the cooler, *i.e.* relatively Nordic and schizothyme, part and the warmer, relatively Alpine and cyclothyme belt.

At present the centre of gravity for political talent and commercial-technical development lies in the zone of cooler temperament (England, north Germany and north America —which is, of course, largely Nordic). On the other hand, the centre of greatest artistic culture lies now, as in former times, in the warmer, more Alpine zone (south and central Germany, upper and middle Italy, and France), as statistics show. Moreover, that artistic culture is of a kind appealing directly to the senses, objective, demanding an immediate emotional response and a warmth of temperament. Between these two extreme wings, stand the more thoughtful, rationalistic forms of culture, expressed mainly in the activities of poets and philosophers. It is true that these thrive in both zones, from England and north Germany southwards to central Italy, but there are certain significant differences between the parts. The schizothyme members of this group, namely the philosophers and tragic dramatists, are essentially more strongly represented in the northern and middle racial belts, whilst towards the south, in Italy and among the more cyclothyme German stocks, they fade out rapidly. Locke, Hume, Descartes, Kant, Herder, Herbart and Schopenhauer derived from the northern zone, as did also Shakespeare, Corneille, Voltaire, Kleist and Hebbel. Conversely, the classical countries of art and music —Italy and the more hypomanic peoples of south Germany —show only sporadic, isolated cases of philosophers (G. Bruno) and geniuses of tragic drama (Grillparzer).

This constitutional difference of endowment between the more Nordic and the more Alpine sections of the zone of intermixture, is as tangible in the statistical presentation of the ancestry of geniuses of recent times as it is in the geographical distribution of Gothic and Renaissance-Baroque culture.

Now each of these zones has an anomalous portion, geographically small but culturally important. Within the southern zone, the Swabian area is different from the rest not only in religion, but in many other manifestations, notably its greater production of philosophers and dramatic geniuses, and its lesser talent in music. It clearly belongs more to the zone of cooler temperament. Conversely, within the Nordic belt, the Netherlands-Flanders area stands out as a small island of eminent talent in painting. Yet, in both cases, the anomalousness concerns only a part of the total endowments, for the Swabian area shares with the rest of the Alpine zone an unusual talent in painting and architecture, whilst Holland clearly belongs to the cooler zone in its Protestant religion and political disposition.

In both areas one might have deduced this partial anomalousness from the racial map. Würtemberg, and especially the old Würtemberg Protestant area around the Neckar, whence most of the philosophers and poets in question are derived, has a strong Nordic ingredient. This intrusion into the valleys of the Main and Neckar of Nordic blood (Günther) corresponds to the old path of migration of the Germanic tribes, and can be readily seen, for example, in the cephalic indexes on the map of Deniker and Fischer. The more Nordic area thus revealed, appears as a narrow, elongated wedge, penetrating along the Main and Neckar valleys far into the Alpine regions. Similarly there seems to be a strongly Alpine racial island in the Netherlands. I quote Günther : " The downward gradient for the Nordic race, *i.e.* its decline from racial purity, is much more rapid in passing from the north to the south of Holland than in the corresponding transition in Germany. We are inclined, in Germany, to regard Holland as being much more Nordic than it really is." Günther then proceeds to enumerate a series of islands of Alpine population, a good number of which lie right in the middle of the Netherlands area and are " in view of the northerly position of Holland, quite exceptional." To these smaller areas we must add the large, Alpine Walloon region in Belgium, which treads closely upon them.

It is remarkable, and perhaps of great importance for racial theory, that we find three places within German-speaking territory at which there is an incredibly disproportionate concentration of genius. Mainly they are places where a special type of genius occurs frequently in a very limited area ; where, statistically expressed, there is exceptional density of genius. These three regions are : Saxony (with the parts of Thuringia and Silesia which border on it), Swabia and the Netherlands. In every case these will be found to be spots where different racial zones pass immediately, and with exceptional abruptness, one into the other. Saxony lies hard between densely Alpine Bohemia and the strongly Nordic provinces of Prussia. The Netherlands show, according to Günther, a rapid ' decline from purity ' of the Nordic race ; and in Würtemberg the Nordic wedge of the Neckar projects sharply into an Alpine region. Thus it is possible to consider this display of genius as a product of blood mixture, similar to that which occurred in the Italian Renaissance or in ancient Greece by intermarriage of the sharply distinguished Nordic nobility with a native population of different racial origin.

In both of the latter cases the blossoming of genius apparently took place simultaneously with a break-up of social classes, and the collapse of social stratification was virtually a disruption of racial exclusiveness. Here we are laying emphasis not only, with Sommer and Reibmayr, on the rôle of racial fusion as the soil of genius, but also on the sharpness of the distinction between the fusing elements and on the effect of the social situation in which inter-marriage takes place.

Within the Nordic-Alpine intermixture zone we frequently find special zones which are of some interest because they represent concentrated talent developing in some particular direction. These special zones show, in the first place, a development of the general gifts of the racial endowment ; but they also evidence the effects of national and family inbreeding. We find, for example, that the greater part of creative musical talent in Germany has arisen in that circumscribed stock of population which runs in a semi-circle round the central Bohemian core of the Alpine race and stretches thence towards the Alps. The main body of German musical genius comes from Saxony-Thuringia (Bach, Handel, Schumann, Richard Wagner), north-eastern Bavaria (Gluck, Reger) and Austria (Haydn, Mozart, Schubert, Weber, Liszt, Bruckner, Hugo Wolf). For musical genius, *i.e.* the capacity to express spiritual profundities in music, descent from the Alpine race has clearly, up to the present, been the decisive factor. The history of music in Europe has been made, in its essentials, solely by the three nations with a strong Alpine component : Germany, Italy and France. And among these it is the regions with the softer, hypomanic temperament which hold the first place. Here stand Italy, Austria and Saxony : the musical culture produced by them in the last few centuries is a unique creation among all peoples and through all times. In other nations and races musical endowment is widespread and freely distributed, but nowhere up to the present has there been that soaring, monumental growth of musical master-pieces which has occurred in the regions where the Alpine racial ingredients predominate. That Alpine racial origin presents the most important factor in musical talent is proved further by the fact that zones occupied by pure Nordic or pure Mediterranean people (Spain) fall furthest of all behind the Alpine admixture areas we have considered. Many Nordic race areas, such as England and the north-west German provinces, are notorious for their lack of musical productivity (Frisia non cantat). From such ex-pressive geographical quantitative proofs it must be accepted that a certain dash of Alpine blood is always present in musical geniuses of the Alpine-Nordic zone, even if the physical characteristics of this race are sometimes difficult to detect in individual cases.

Poetic-philosophical endowment is found in Germany in two centres of great density : Saxony (with its Thuringian and Silesian neighbouring parts) and Würtemberg. To the first place belong, among others, Luther, Leibnitz, Lessing, Eichendorff, Fichte, Schleiermacher, Otto Ludwig, and Nietzsche ; to the latter, Wieland, Schiller, Hölderlin, Uhland, Mörike, Hegel and Schelling. In poetic achieve-ments the Alsace-Lorraine area also plays a part, with Keller, Meyer and Gotthelf. In addition to the really great names, there are many smaller names in the history of literature thickly scattered in both these areas. Saxony, in consequence of the coincidence of musical with poetic-philosophic talent, is quite the richest area in genius in all

Germany. Most of the remaining names in this group of talented men come from the northern strip of Germany, but they are there more thinly distributed and sporadically arranged, *e.g.* Klopstock, Kant, Herder, Herbart, Schopenhauer, Kleist, Hebbel, Droste-Hülshoff, Storm and Fontane. On the other hand the more hypomanic stocks of the Alpine zone, namely, those in Austria, Bavaria, and Franconia (around the Rhine and the Main), make a very weak contribution to this field of talent. In the whole vast area the only relief is found in the two great names of Goethe and Grillparzer, of whom the first has strong genealogical relations with the people of Thuringia-Saxony and Würtemberg. But then, there is compensation for this when one thinks that the greatest focus of musical genius lies in Austria and of plastic art in Franconia. In the realm of Germanic speech, the plastic and graphic arts concentrate themselves mostly in the Netherlands and Franconia (Dürer, Grünewald, Cranach, Peter Vischer, Riemenschneider, Feuerbach). In the second rank come the Austro-Bavarian (Leibl, Lenbach, Spitzweg, Schwind) and Swabian-Alsatian areas (famous for its schools of painting and architecture from the Middle Ages to the Baroque period, and for the names of Holbein, Böcklin and Thoma). At this point we encounter another fact of great racial significance. Just as the Nordic Neckar region clearly held the lead in the southern regions for poetic-philosophic talent, so it relinquishes it to the Alpine Swabian-Alsatian area where the plastic arts are concerned. We need only mention Ulm, Augsburg, Vorarlberg (Baroque), Switzerland and the southern Black Forest region. Old Würtemberg has produced neither a famous painter nor a great musician.

Military and political talent of the old stamp we find

most strongly concentrated in the nobility, which, in all nations of the Nordic-Alpine zone, is predominantly Nordic. The centre of gravity in these activities has moved somewhat to the north since the Middle Ages, so that to-day we find the greatest political-military endowment, without a doubt, in England, north Germany and France. On the whole, ability in this direction declines, in all nations in the racial fusion zone, as we pass from north to south, a fact which clearly demonstrates the relation of such talent to the Nordic race. However, 'military-political' talent is no unified psychological entity. Modern politics and economics differ essentially in their methods and goals from the politics of the old nobility. In opposition to the stiff and unalterable ideology of the old school, they demand leaders with more intellectual elasticity, subtle intuition, broad-minded spirit and penetrating, realistic insight. In short, strong hypo-manic dispositional factors are required, such as the Nordic race only sparingly possesses, but which, together with the necessary hardness and consistency, can be found in many of the complicated Nordic alloys with Alpine elements.

Here also, then, the admixture of alien blood, acts as a desirable ferment, bringing out the specific racial talents, whereas relatively pure races, after long inbreeding, mani-festly acquire a certain petrifaction of their talents, a certain narrowness and uselessness—as Reibmayr has already recognised. Hence the political centre of gravity among the Nordic peoples does not lie in the parts of greatest racial purity. In Great Britain, for example, it lies, not in Scotland, but in southern England. Within the German Empire it lies, not in the north-west corner, but in the more easterly parts : Prussia. We can probably bring into line here, as the converse analogous case, the fact that the

G

peak of musical talent does not lie in the purest Alpine race centre in Bohemia, but round the periphery of that region.

From these comparisons of the geographical distribution of genius, we obtain on most points, a decidedly clear picture of the intellectual dispositions of the Nordic and Alpine races. Moreover it has proved to be a picture which remains true whether we approach it from one side or the other. To one race belongs the centre of gravity in philosophy and drama ; to the other, with its emphatic artistic temperament, has been given the greater endowment in music and the plastic arts. Yet, as far as the facts go, we are only able to say : within the zone of racial admixture, this part has, in the past, made such and such contributions, and that part has manifested other endowments. We cannot assert that the pure races would have attained such levels, or even have proceeded in such directions, separately. Indeed, we can with greater probability suppose that the racial fusion, with its fermentative and enriching effects, played an essential part in those developments. We must adopt this supposition because the region of racial intermixture shows a much stronger production of genius than the geographical zones of relatively pure race ; and again because the most outstanding individual geniuses are rarely pure race types and do not always correspond to the racial type of their area.

Into the question of the rise of ' sub-races ' by continued inbreeding within established areas of political and linguistic unity, with its alleged production of national and regional types, we cannot enter in any detail. But it seems possible to suppose that the nations formed by Nordic-Alpine fusion, just like the children of corresponding marriages, are distinctly new individuals, distinguished not merely by the percentage proportions of intermixture, but by a unique

combination and selection of the parental race characteristics, which gives them an individual stamp.

The mixture of Nordic and Alpine races has provided
us with an especially clear example of the way in which
the hybridisation of partly dissimilar races, by compensating
and supporting the characters of each component, can give
rise to a complete and vital civilisation, *i.e.* to a series of
populations constantly breeding a sufficiency of men of
genius. The example is also the only one concerning which
a sufficiently sound and comprehensive amount of statistical
material, in the form of anthropological and historical facts,
is available as a basis for really scientific judgments. One
may assume, with some probability, that the rise of lofty
civilisations, blossoming with genius, at other times and in
other races and nations, was caused by a similar biological
process of cross-breeding. For in individual human biology
too, suitable cross-breeding gives rise to richly-developed
' hybrids ' who easily outgrow the parental types from which
they have sprung. The breeding of genius is thus assimilated
to the same process which, in specialist biology, is known
as the ' luxuriation ' of hybrids. Hence highly-developed
civilisations are usually produced within a definite time
interval after the migrations of peoples and the invasions of
conquering tribes which have gradually mixed themselves
with the native populations.

From this observation arises very frequently the erroneous
conclusion that the immigrating or invading race, as such,
has brought genius with it. Such a conclusion plays an
important part in the train of reasoning which leads to the
apotheosis of the Nordic race and to its present lofty position
in popular estimation. Such an error can be easily avoided
if one takes the trouble to study the same race in its purest

possible condition, in its original home, where it will be found in vigorous, industrious, but narrow and unenterprising pursuit of old occupations, agricultural customs and traditions, just like any other capable race. And even a great restlessness, manifested in migration and conquest, can only be regarded as a normal demonstration of vitality and valour, such as occurs in all healthy and unexhausted tribes among the most varied races. The masterful characters of a conquering people can be observed quite as easily in the history of the Mongolian, Indian and Arabian peoples as in the old Teutons. Tribes and peoples that have been constantly engaged in migration and conquest are not necessarily 'superior and heroic' peoples, but mainly, and in the first place, tribes situated in northern and desert lands, *i.e.* poor, climatically-unbearable, sterile habitats, which drive them ceaselessly into efforts to break through into rich, settled, civilised areas. Neither is it right to call the invading people the 'superior' people and the indigenous population the 'slave race'. Romantic, sounding epithets of that kind should be strenuously avoided in such a difficult and complex subject. Instead, one must first recognise that the outcome of any of these attempts at conquest is solely dependent upon the degree of ripeness at which the civilisation of the attacked people stands. And this life-phase of a cultural community has nothing whatever to do with the vigour and capability of the native race which supports it, as Spengler has already very beautifully shown. If the civilisation of the established peoples happens to be just at its period of most powerful development, the attackers will be repulsed and annihilated, without reference to whether they are Nordic (Celts, Teutons) or Mongolian in race. But should they fall upon a decaying civilisation, then the assault will succeed—and a racial fusion will supervene, which, granted a favourable degree of comparability and fitness in the qualities of the two races, will lead to a new civilisation and a renewed production of genius. And that blossoming will take place, not in the original home of the invading people, but away in the conquered country, where hybridisation is occurring.

From this it is an easy step to the supposition that the natural law which appears to hold in regard to the rise and fall of great civilisations, and which has been so fully expounded by Spengler, is based biologically on the alternation of inbreeding and cross-breeding and that this conditions many of the manifestations appearing in the social life of classes, nations and races. But notice that both in the examples and in the general discussion we have been referring to a pair of thoroughly inbred races as the units of fusion, *i.e.* stocks which through long residence in a given area, accompanied by intermarriage of blood relatives, have each attained to a firmly impressed hereditary type, characterised by definite groups of physical and mental peculiarities. Moreover, the degree of similarity and difference between the peoples has been just about the same as that which is normally recognised as necessary for the production of vigorous hybrids in animals and plants. Reibmayr has already made it quite clear that whereas the crossing of talented, inbred stocks may lead to genius, the intermarriage of unselected currents of population, coming together by chance, as happens to a considerable extent in big, cosmopolitan cities, never does so, but leads in the opposite direction ('blood chaos'). Metropoli require men of genius, but they do not themselves produce them, as can be easily proved by statistics.

Hybridisation can come to pass through peaceful changes or through warlike invasion, through the breaking-down of impenetrable class walls and from a number of similar social processes.   In a definite time after such mixture of bloods, there appears a strong crop of genius, and therewith a period of advanced civilisation, which lasts just as long as the basic biological effects persist.   The 'dying-out' of a lofty culture may result from one of two biological processes. In the first place, the propagation of such a civilised community may continue without any external hindrance. Then there will enter again, after the exhaustion of the spiritual ferment due to hybridisation, a period of stable inbreeding, and therewith a steady national existence accompanied by a certain stiffening and fixity (Chinese type).   In the second contingency, the instincts of propagation may become impaired by the complexity of civilisation. A rapid depopulation of the best elements will then lead to a catastrophic collapse (Late Roman Empire type).   In both cases there remains the biological possibility of calling forth a new culture and a new dawn of genius by causing the original, resident race to blend with another, suitably chosen, stock.   Theoretically this process could be repeated without limit.   Long-lived ancient civilisations, such as those of Egypt and Assyria-Babylon, seem to have owed their constantly renewed vitality within the same environment, to repeated cross-breedings of the kind described.   This theoretically-unlimited capacity of resuscitation possessed by the culture of any country, rests in the end upon the astonishingly tenacious life of the original native race, which, within the short span of time occupied by historical eras, seems to have neither youth nor age.   It goes on growing as does the simple grass and herbage of the country-side, untroubled by the coming and going of those magnificent hybrid garden flowers—the men of genius, the great city civilisations, the political powers—which have arisen by interbreeding with them.

For that reason it is not sound to compare the life-course of a civilisation with the birth, growth and death of a single individual. Individuality as a guiding principle is being carried too far if it leads anyone to think of any particular culture period as something of unique value, beyond comparison and incapable of being repeated. The civilisation of the Italian Renaissance is something different from the civilisation of antiquity, but it is only partially and conditionally different. A new hybridisation of the same native race produced it ; an element of the same attitude to life linked them together ; and they possessed a common store of intellectual riches and spiritual traditions. Perhaps, from the standpoint of remote peoples and times, the Graeco-Roman culture, modern civilisation, and the blossomings and fadings of civilisation that may stretch through the next millennium, will all appear as a single, self-contained cultural unit. But if our principles are true, what of the Peruvian civilisation and ancient inhabitants of Mexico ? Possibly the ancient Indian population will continue to grow, as it has done, in the old places, until no drop of blood from white immigrants is any longer discernible. But on the other hand they may form with those immigrants a race of vigorous hybrids, who will bring forth a rich Inca civilisation, different from and yet related, as the Renaissance was to antiquity, to the intellectual spirit and racial mood of the ancient culture. Who knows when civilisation may begin to flower again vigorously in the deserts of Babylon or remote Arabia, in Egypt or China ? It blossoms again and perhaps yet again in the ancient places—who knows ?   And what is there really within such apparently great perspectives as ' Western Civilisation ' and ' Decline ' ?   Life has a vast stride and knows nothing of our tiny historical epochs, our separate civilisations and our tiny individualities.   Above all, it pays no attention, in the great things, to any ' I '. Life blooms and withers and blooms again, and the goal of this blossoming and fading—we do not know.   There may still be hundreds of hybrid blooms waiting to spring from us through the centuries, each different from and yet similar to, the others.   The West has still countless civilisations and men of genius to hope for and expect in its decline—if it believes that civilisation and genius are things worthy of hope and expectation.

PART TWO
PATTERNS

SIXTH CHAPTER

Spiritual Periodicity

The Artist of Life

No form of mental and spiritual activity, especially if it be the creative force of genius, flows evenly and constantly through the whole course of life. Rather, in the intellectual life of great men, is there usually a peculiar wave-like course, a coming and going, a welling-up of passionate excitement and an exhausted sinking down again. A genius suddenly gripped by inspiration, finds himself, as an artist, swept up into an overwhelming and varied productivity of pictures and music, or, as a scientist, overpowered by surprising flashes of insight and a rich grasp of relations. He works feverishly, day and night, through weeks and months, to give his ideas shape and form, thereafter to find himself, perhaps for a long time, barren of ideas, incapable of activity and fruitless in execution. This periodic undulation is a definite characteristic peculiarity of much of the work of genius—of really productive mental work in contrast to the reproductive, daily, bread-and-butter activities of the average man, which are regularly supplied from the wells of habit and tradition and unfold themselves evenly from day to day.

And yet this periodicity in the creativeness of genius, is no remote metaphysical wonder, which only appears in the highest spheres of pure intellect ; it is much more the reverse, a token of how closely the loftiest flights of mind are bound down to the ordinary cosmic processes, to the interrelations of mind and body and the laws determining the course of Nature around us. Through the movements of the earth and the planets all life is made periodic. The seasons, the changes of the moon, day and night, divide up the life of all animals and plants into patterns of work and rest. The fluctuations of the sexual life, constitutes in man, the most important biological basis for the differentiations in the course of his intellectual life. The storm and stress of puberty, the profound emotional disturbances at the time of the change of life, the retrospection of old age and the slight continuous changes of outlook which the seasonal variations condition in our instinctive sensibilities—all these are effects of the acutest significance for the understanding of human feelings and activities, but specially of the creative acts of genius.

But here again, arise great individual differences. The stronger a man is in his mental construction, the less he will be disturbed by the fluctuation of surrounding cosmos and his own bodily resonance, the less his spiritual life will be under their influence, the better he will be able to resist them. It is precisely this steadiness which must be regarded as the token of a healthy, normal mentality.

The average, robust human being, soons learns to direct his mental processes in such a way that they obey him steadily in all phases of his mental periodicity. He gets through his work as well in the morning as in the evening. Neither is he diverted by the joy of spring or thrown into discord by the cold miasma of winter.

Conversely, it is precisely in certain groups of mentally abnormal persons that this periodicity of the emotional life is found in its most exaggerated forms. Whenever the mental disposition is very sensitive and plastic in certain directions, there the periodic influences of body and general environment will find a much more pronounced resonance.

There exists indeed, as we know, a very widespread form of mental disease, which is called periodic or circular insanity, and which is connected with an inherited disposition commonly designated 'manic-depressive'. Manic-depressive persons, not only react with especial readiness to the environmental influences outlined above, but are also subject, quite apart from this rhythm, to a regular periodic fluctuation between an inhibited melancholic depression in the depressive phase and a gay, lively urge to expression in the other, manic phase.

This manic-depressive or circular disposition is found in all degrees of strength from the slightest, barely perceptible, periodic fluctuation in the emotional life of the healthy man to the profoundest melancholia and raving mania. It is found among men of genius, indeed, it occasionally forms the family psychosis of such men, occurring again and again here and there through the generations of talented artistic families. The fact can be more easily appreciated if we observe how closely the manic group of symptoms, with its overflowing vitality, its wild, kaleidoscopic flight of ideas and its creative energy, resembles the productivity period in the life of genius. Conversely we perceive how nearly the melancholic phase of circular insanity runs parallel to the spiritual dearth and barrenness, the feelings of despondency and despair, which reside with so many men of genius in the interludes between their periods of creative work.

From this standpoint we may look at the life of Goethe. so closely analysed by Möbius, whose presentation we have frequently followed. Here we soon notice that the Olympic calm and detachment which superficial observers were so ready to ascribe to him are in reality scarcely to be discovered, that his moods were constantly changing and that long intervals of spiritual aridity were interrupted in a regular cycle by shorter periods of general intellectual, erotic and poetic stimulation.

When young people occasionally get a fit of amorousness and verse-making, that is no symptom of a periodic or circular constitution. For that reason we will begin, in order to be quite clear, with Goethe's later life. Goethe himself very characteristically remarked : ' The man of genius experiences a repetition of adolescence, whereas other people are only youthful once.' In the last years of his life Goethe complained that work, which had previously always been play to him, was a thing to which he now had to force himself. '' Only the summer of 1831,'' reported Vogel, his physician, '' was an exception in this respect,'' and Goethe often asserted during that time that he had never been so disposed to intellectual work, especially of a productive kind, for the previous thirty years. Actually there reigned in Goethe's nature during the year 1830–31 a peculiar excitement which evidenced itself in great activity and a lively reactiveness. Out of his letters to Zelter there speaks a positively feverish eagerness. In this period Goethe completed his biography and at last put the finishing touches to *Faust*.

If we pass from this last upward swing to a time about seven years before, we encounter in the years 1821–23 a highly remarkable period of Goethe's life, which sharply interrupts the peaceful course of life of the seventy-four-year-old man. The negligent manner of the dignified, rather stiff official began now to become young and tender again ; he fell in love with the nineteen-year-old Ulrike von Levetzow.

At Marienbad and Karlsbad he shows himself to be gay, full of gallantry and peculiarly amorously stimulated. Music moves him to tears ; he has consoling dreams ; his letters have a positively ecstatic tone, he asserts that he finds himself in a state of bodily and mental well-being such as he has not known for many years. In fact his love for the nineteen-year-old Ulrike brought this seventy-four-year-old man to thoughts of marriage. The grand-duke had to step forward as a match-maker and Goethe himself wrote letters which came very near to what in normal life would be called a proposal. On his way home in September he wrote the ' Elegy '. " Dejection, woe, reproach and weariness burden the oppressive air."

At that point his spirits swing into a phase of profound depression. He sits at home sorely disconsolate, bursts into tears, and tortures himself with hypochondriac troubles, until at last, under Zelter's loving care, he gradually makes a recovery.

If now we again take a step seven years backward from this last poetic love, we encounter, in the year 1814–15 a no less peculiar island in the course of Goethe's spiritual life. That is the period of the *Westöstlichen Divan* and the love of Marianne von Willemer. The serious, regulated industry of the government official, of the scientist, the collector and the critic, which characterised the dignified, precise mental presence of the ageing Goethe is here unexpectedly interrupted by a kind of renewed adolescence. A lively poetry of the heart begins to burst forth as from a bubbling spring. On the 21st of July 1814 Goethe writes the first song. By the end of August thirty poems have already appeared, until in May 1815 the first hundred poems are complete. Then follows his love for Marianne von

Willemer, and in the *Suleika Lyrics* Goethe attains to new
heights. Still to-day in some of those verses his passionate
eagerness is borne down to us.

> Nur dies Herz, es ist von Dauer,
> Schwillt in jugendlichstem Flor;
> Unter Schnee und Nebelschauer
> Rast ein Ätna Dir hervor.
>
> Du beschämst wie Morgenröte
> Jener Gipfel ernste Wand.
> Und noch einmal fühlet Hatem
> Frühlingshauch und Sommerbrand.
>
> Schenke her! Noch eine Flasche!
> Diesen Becher bring ich ihr!
> Findet sie ein Haüfchen Asche,
> Sagt sie: der verbrannte mir.

A powerful, passionate temperament and a completely
youthful freshness come to expression in many of these
lyrics. They continue to live still in the musical settings of
Schubert and Hugo Wolf, whereas the numerous more
serious and significant poems of art and philosophy appearing
in the surrounding years have faded for our feelings even
though not for our intellectual interest. Always it is the
lyrics out of Goethe's stimulated period which alone live
on. Goethe himself felt quite clearly that the ability to
write poetry came upon him like a fever, that when the
moment decreed it he must write poetry and that when
the excitement had run its course the well of song dried
up again. In the arid period later he himself said to Ecker-
mann: ' The Lieder des Divans have no point of contact
with me at all. Both that which is oriental and that which
is passionate in them have ceased to live in me any longer.
It is like a cast-off snake skin that has been left lying in
the path.'

One is naturally tempted to say : love called forth the lyrics ; for whenever Goethe became acquainted with any women his feelings awoke in him poetic fire. The explanation misses the mark. Goethe had always had pretty young ladies and women around him. But he only fell in love at given times. And then the chosen one had no need to have outstanding qualities. It is also significant for the periodicity of Goethe's mental life that, when once his inclinations began to murmur from within he became passionately attached to several within a relatively short period. Almost all the people Goethe loved are, from the point of view of time, grouped closely at long intervals : Lotte in Wetzlar and Maximiliane la Roche, Lili Schönemann and Frau von Stein, the lady of Milan and Christiana Vulpius, Minna Herzlieb and Silvia von Ziegesar.

However, the appearance of the *Westöstlichen Divan* offers the clearest proof that feminine personalities were not in themselves the cause of Goethe's access of poetic activity. It shows that, on the contrary, the excitement already present caused him to fall in love with such women as appeared in his immediate circle at the time of inward stimulation. With the *Westöstlichen Divan* itself the source of lyric poetry begins to flow again, unexpectedly and without any gradual onset, after a pause of many years. The excitement, the general feeling of vitality, has already been present for some months before Goethe comes into contact with Marianne von Willemer. She is the object of his love because he has been in a phase of poetic excitement, not the converse. Had he met her about 1811 instead of 1814 she would presumably have left him cold. And it is especially significant that from 1816 onwards, after the period of excitement had died away, he never saw Marianne

H

again and gave up a projected journey to see her, on account of some trivial difficulty. Only in the next period of stimulation, 1823, during the time he was in love with Ulrike von Levetzow did he begin suddenly, on the homeward journey, to write to Marianne. As he himself said, he thought of her when " I became once more full of turmoil."

As we have already seen, the periods of excitement with Goethe lasted about two years whilst the quieter less vital periods in between continued usually for about seven years. If we now go back seven years we do in fact come upon another period of rejuvenescence in the years 1807–08 with the dual love for Minchen Herzlieb and Silvia von Ziegesar. This period saw the birth of the Sonnets and the work on elective affinities continued to grow ; the Diary arose. The good, creative mood lasted on into the winter. But from 1809 onwards the usual dryness reigned once more. After a time of ill-health there began suddenly, during a cure at Karlsbad, an onset of general excitement and therewith of amorous feelings. Whilst busied in lively poetic creation during the autumn he became strongly attracted to Minna Herzlieb. This attraction gave way in the following summer, after a well-spent winter, to an intimate relation with Silvia.

Now although Goethe's middle age falls thus into four regularly outcropping periods of excitement, 1801–08, 1814–15, 1822–23, 1830–31 the wave-like motion is somewhat obscured in the two preceding decades of his life. The prime of Goethe's life from 1789–1807 is the time of his greatest spiritual health and balance. Yet it was poetically the least productive time of his life and the poems which have remained alive until to-day derive in by far the greatest number either from his early life up to the Italian tour or, as with the *Westöstlichen Divan* from his old age. We may recall the peculiar spiritual desolation and loneliness which dominated Goethe's life for several years after his return from Italy and which was interrupted only by the appearance of Schiller. It is the time of spiritless stylistic poems, of interest in art, of wandering in antiquity, of work constantly renewed and neglected, and of petty, ineffective dramas of a day. It is a popular assumption by writers on literature, but an assumption which brings no illumination, that after his return from Italy the narrow life of Weimar influenced his life so evilly that he remained for many years poetically sterile. A poet, when the spirit is with him, will create poetry in the most miserable, unheated attic. That Goethe in the relatively interesting and spiritually rich Society of Weimar was prevented for many long years from making poetry is hard to believe.

Whosoever is inwardly intellectually stimulated will find rich and interesting experience in the most banal little provincial town, but when the inner drive is lacking the most brilliant circles will simply bore him. It was not any dissatisfaction with his immediate neighbourhood which caused Goethe to feel ill-tempered and isolated ; it was rather the absence of the right mood in himself which prevented his receiving any stimulation from his environment.

Schiller had already been living for years in Goethe's neighbourhood. In 1788–89 he was in Weimar itself and sought in every way to attain to a communion of feeling with Goethe. Their acquaintances spared no trouble to bring about that happy state of affairs for them. It was all in vain. Goethe persistently withdrew himself with distinct coolness. He gave no sign of having noticed the appearance of *Don Carlos ;* Schiller's poems found no approval from him and the work on ' Grace and Dignity ' even awoke his spite. And then at last after some years, without anyone really knowing why, a complete change occurred. A letter from Schiller received a warmer response, in which there was even talk of friendship. And immediately there are cordial relationships and a fullness of lively intercourse. The way in which this friendship arose after years of aversion is so remarkable that one cannot be too astonished at it. Let us reckon now from the last-mentioned period of animation in Goethe's life in the year 1807–08. Going back twice seven years we come to the year 1794. 1794 is the year in which Goethe suddenly developed his friendship for Schiller. With this simple arithmetical sum one of the most critical and enigmatic points in the history of Goethe's spiritual development is cleared up. After a seven-year period of inanition and general fretfulness Goethe again becomes lively in a hypomanic sense, productive, sociable, ready to give and ready to take love and friendship. Instead of love for a woman, which usually gripped him with unfailing regularity at these times, he developed on this occasion his most profound and intimate friendship with another man. And just as the beloved woman on other occasions had been a stimulus to poetic productivity so now did his spiritual friend. It was in the succeeding years that " Hermann and Dorothea " was given shape.

Undoubtedly the entrance of Schiller into Goethe's life brought to bear a powerful external influence and one which maintained its significance more than such influences generally did, out into the period beyond the actual interval of animation. But the reason for this factor entering at all ; the reason for Goethe ever becoming friendly with Schiller after he had disliked him for so many years, is a matter which can be explained only by a biological analysis not a literary-historical one.

Meanwhile we have overlooked the period of stimulation which should fall between 1794 and 1808. It is indeed not very clearly marked, though not insignificant. Actually some important parts of *Faust* were written at this time ; the promenade, the Easter scene and the second monologue, *i.e.* precisely the parts which in poetic power stand nearest to the *Urfaust* of Goethe's youth.

So much for the years of Goethe's prime. On considering finally the period of his youth we notice two soaring moments of climax. There is, to begin with, the great period of vital genius which began at the end of his studentship at Strasbourg, reached its summit in the year 1773 with the novel *Werther* and his love for Lili Schönemann and then gradually declined into the elegant stillness of the poet of *Iphigeneia* and *Tasso*, finally to lose itself in the Goethe of Weimar. In these years Goethe's spiritual life was in stormy movement, whirled up and down between the maddest joy of living and downcast thoughts of suicide. Passionate love and feverish eagerness in poetic creation held him in constant activity. One youthful love dissolved itself in another, from Frederika in Sessenheim to Lotte in Wetzlar and Lili Schönemann.

Götz, Faust and Werther are only a few of the great pictures which his imagination at that time was constantly and inexhaustibly creating. It is the time when Goethe lived most eagerly, loved most fervently, and created the most immortal poetry.

The other peak is formed by the Italian tour in the years 1786–88 in which Goethe's youth both inwardly and outwardly came to an end. Poetically and in his love to

Frau von Stein, Goethe had gradually drifted to a dead point. His great works, *Egmont* and *Elpenor*, stood still, *Faust* resisted all attempts to carry it forward, *Tasso*, after two unsatisfying acts, was broken off, *Wilhelm Meister* was postponed. Suddenly in September 1780 Goethe, the state official and privy councillor, disappeared. He vanished without a sign, like a thief in the night, to Italy. There he gave himself up to the gayest and most untrammelled life for nearly two years, fell in love, travelled, made the most beautiful poems and at last returned to Weimar, where he fell in love just once more, with a flower girl. This girl he married in the end, and finally became once more the worthy man of duty that he remained for the greater part of his later life.

Let us seek to look at this episode as it really is, stripped of the phrases of conventional hero-worship and viewed by the sober, respectable citizen. Imagine to yourself that a certain councillor X suddenly leaves all his ministerial duties, his documents and portfolios and, without any leave of absence, disappears in hot haste to Italy, spends two years in a life of pleasure and finally marries a working girl from a none too respectable family. Suppose that both before and after this interlude, he showed himself a good, solid, common-sense, industrious man. What should we say about it ? The usual literary-historical attempts at explanation are once again entirely unsatisfactory for they fail to realise what is cause and what is effect. Now let us count backwards once more seven years from that strange beginning of the friendship with Schiller and we shall find at once another illustration of that regular wave-like motion in Goethe's emotional life ; first a growing intellectual desiccation, a poetic sterility, an increasing crossness tending to isolation, which in a few years reaches an overstrained state. And then suddenly an explosion of impulsive, daring acts which lead to restless activity, a lusty urge to live, erotic stimulation and the creative fertility of genius. Finally the excitement dies down again to quiet, even-flowing moderation. That is Goethe's life curve and at the same time the typical life curve of the manic-depressive or circular personality.

Passing twice seven years backward we arrive at the year of *Werther*, 1773, the summit of the great period of animation which stamped the youthful Goethe as a genius. That period, because of its coincidence with the turmoil of adolescence, was especially deep and persistent. The intermediate terminus, 1780–81, is recognisable to a finer analysis as a time of earnest, solemn, tragic mood which developed an erotic and poetic animation visible in the letters to Frau von Stein.

The last step in our backward journey leads to the year 1767, to the first circular oscillation of the eighteen-year-old Goethe, to the passionate love for Kätchen Schönkopf and the mad Leipzig student days, followed in Frankfort by a strange depression of the emotions accompanied by hypo-chondriac illusions and pietistic moods.

These were the youthful, boisterous years. The older Goethe wore the mask of an artist of human life, the assumed calmness of a prince of poets. All that was an ' overcompensation ', a great stylish gesture, behind which all the pain and joy of life accumulated and was with difficulty dispersed. Only those who use art in life—can be artists of life. Behind it all one can detect the gentle but inexorable pull of the currents of his spiritual periodicity, the darkly perceived undercurrent of his being. But even if one wished it he could not overlook the hereditary connection of this seemingly beneficial process with the tragic family inheritance which annihilated Goethe's relatives in four generations. One is bound to see the eccentric father, the insane sister, the precipitous degeneration of Goethe's children and grand-children. An uncertain, dangerous inheritance, of which the poet's own cyclic disposition was only a fortunate limiting case.

Goethe's father was a marked eccentric who followed no occupation and was the victim finally of an arterio-sclerotic mental disturbance. Of Goethe's five brothers and sisters not one was in any sense physically or mentally robust. Four died of disease in the earliest years, a younger brother who lived until his sixth year was mentally degenerate, slow and abnormally wilful. The only child beside Goethe that grew up—his sister Cornelie—was an unhappily-endowed, thoroughly pathological personality and at times clearly insane. Although in many physical peculiarities the very image of her brilliant brother, she was constantly sickly, ugly in bodily proportions and with sharp, protruding, ill-set features. Her love life was stunted, for she seemed capable neither of exciting love nor of giving it. She was, as her brother remarked, an indefinable being, the strangest mixture of severity and soft-heartedness, self-will and sub-missiveness, and withal earnest, stiff and strangely unlovable. One might have said of her, remarked Goethe, that she was without faith, hope or charity. The picture which her nearest relatives draw of her is entirely without consoling features. Every kind of mental excitement made her ill. Her emotional condition was disturbed and heavy. She was constantly dissatisfied with herself and the world. She wanted to be merry and yet had not a single consoling illusion. She thirsted for love but rejected every tender advance, and though she wished to open her heart she repelled everyone by her sharpness and bitterness. After her first delivery of a child in the year 1774 she became insane. For nearly two years she remained profoundly melancholic, rooted to one spot, incapable of any activity and tortured herself with constant fears and terrible insane illusions. After a short happier interlude she became incurably ill and died in 1777 only twenty-seven years old.

Goethe's sister would be characterised as a schizoid and strongly depressed personality with episodic attacks of melancholy, and the diseased emotional condition can be easily recognised as a part of the total, hereditary anomalousness of feelings in the Goethe family. Thus a similar disposition to that which, in an evil, diseased form, destroyed the whole life happiness of the sister, served with the brother, in the form of a mild cyclic oscillation of the emotions, as the provider of the richest gifts of feeling and imagination.

The fate of the Goethe family fulfilled itself quickly in the descendants of the poet himself. Of five children only one remained alive ; August Goethe, a diseased and unhappy nature. The neighbourhood called him ' the mad gentleman '. Already in his boyhood he had begun to drink immoderately. His life was a chain of tempestuous attempts at this and that, of failure and unhappiness for which he had himself to blame. Whatsoever he acquired by his goodness of heart, his loyal friendships and his honest striving for a worthy reputation he lost again by his immoderate impulsiveness, his uncertain, disorderly behaviour and his morose ill-temper. In short he manifested the symptoms of a severe hereditary degeneracy, which, in the last years of his life, passed into an emphatic insanity. He died, probably as the result of his dipsomania, whilst travelling in Italy, at the early age of forty-one.

With the two unfortunate sons that he left behind, the house of Goethe died out. The eldest, Walter Wolfgang, of small, weak, crippled physique, was a quiet, repressed, suffering nature who showed no gifts except in his love of music, and who finally died of consumption. The younger, Wolf Goethe, who was poetically talented and of some spiritual greatness, suffered severely with his nerves. He remained taciturn and unstable in emotion, until in later life, dejected and ill, he withdrew himself into isolation. With the death of these two brothers the misery of the Goethe family came to an end.

People are so fond of holding up Goethe as the prototype of powerful intellectual health and balanced harmony of spirit. Goethe's family circle teaches us something quite different. When we see how his brother and sister withered away in their tenderest youth and how the only remaining sister was spared merely to pass away in bitterness, feebleness and gloom, when we see how nearly the poet himself is touched by the same force that ruined his sister, then we can trace the working of real human fate. We can recognise the same family destiny as poisoned also the lives of Beethoven or Michelangelo. We perceive genius at last as the shape of Iphigeneia, as the last bright blossom among the distorted products of a degenerating species. There stands by Goethe a sister, as there stood by Iphigeneia a dark melancholy brother. And we understand the song of the Fates, the symbol of the shining, golden favourite of the gods, dining on cliffs and clouds in abysses of the deep, who to-morrow will swallow up all his Titan offspring.

SEVENTH CHAPTER

Sex and Puberty

The Curves of Life

A MAN to whom research on genius owes a good deal, the clever psychiatrist Möbius, once wrote a short paper under the title " On the weak-mindedness of women ". This article awoke such general indignation that it became a byword. Behind the polemical title and among many one-sided exaggerations there was a sound treatment of some of the problems touching the question of genius, *e.g.* that up till now there has been no women genius in the narrower sense of the term and very few women who have created original values in any field of intellectual endeavour. To this one may object at once that women have never been given equal opportunity in intellectual life, and that in any case their efforts are not properly appreciated owing to long-established prejudice. But, says Möbius quite rightly, have women been prevented from singing and playing the piano ; and why then do they not compose music ? And when they do compose, why do they not compose immortal music ? Möbius went to the trouble to gather together the names of all women composers discoverable in history. In that long register of names we find among the few that mean anything to us, only Clara Schumann who was famous because of her husband, Fanny Mendelssohn remembered because of her brother, and Corona Schröter who became famous through her friend Goethe. And as far as prejudice is concerned it seems that that is negligibly small where pretty musical women are in question.

Nothing can be said, therefore, for the theory that education is to blame. But let us listen again. It is asserted that the subjection of women during thousands of years has led to the inheritance of a stunted spiritual growth which under favourable civilised conditions will quickly disappear again. This is a theory difficult to reconcile with modern biological ideas. For if the mental differences between the male and female sex have arisen in this way over a tremendous space of time and become fixed, then their disappearance would also be a matter of immense intervals of time and hence no object of modern psychological discussion. Therewith we may close the debate as far as the problem of genius is concerned, without, however, wishing to prejudice in any way the feminist position. And we may formulate as an important truth : the complex kind of intellectual creativeness which is recognised sociologically as ' genius ' is very largely confined to the male sex.

The genius of a woman lies in her sons, *i.e.* whatsoever a woman possesses in the way of significant intellectual endowment is in the form of hereditary qualities which can come to full sociological expression in her sons, as is shown by the example of Goethe's mother. Of course there are a few women who perform, not indeed great acts of genius, but yet indubitably original and permanent creative works. In the realm of German poetry there is such a name : Annette von Droste-Hülshoff. But she is straightway perceived to be a very anomalous example. The poems of Droste have actually a harsh, powerful, realistic tone. Their style and language is so rugged and masculine that the verses of many masculine poets appear tender and womanish in comparison. Still more peculiar is the subject-matter. Only in veiled and devious ways does the feminine motif show itself in the choice of subjects, namely in the attention to religion, tradition and the family. On the other hand the whole realm of poetry as it concerns children and love is outside her province and conspicuously lacking in all her creations. Precisely in the place where the emotional life of woman especially and richly unfolds itself, there is with Droste a yawning gap. Her poems seem much more like the songs of a rough huntsman ; they are full of the noise of weapons and the chase, of wild roamings over the moors, of deeds of violence and bloody murder, of armoured prelates and knights, of the gloomy graves of our savage forefathers, over which the grim Germanic gods shake their cloudy hair. These are the tones in her poems which are the most engrossing and the most genuine. Droste-Hülshoff, however, not only feels as a man, but would also like to be one. In one of her Bodensee poems, where she stands in wild weather on the tower, she rises in the concluding stanza to the burning expression of desire : " If I were but a huntsman on open ground, the mere shadow of a soldier, or at least a man. . . ." And from her dream on the ancient cairn she is recalled in the poem by the man-servant with the words ' Sir, it has begun to rain.' This little touch is very characteristic. In order to get into the mood in which her best and most genuine effects were produced she used to have to imagine herself—dressed as a man. It is precisely this predilection for dressing up as a man that betrays the abnormal, contrary, sexual component in psychopathic women. And this mixture of masculine and feminine feelings is found equally in most of the great women of history : Queen Elizabeth of England, Empress Catharine and, especially emphasised, in Queen Christina of Sweden.

We may now compare with Droste-Hülshoff any woman poet who has really sung of spring and love and brought into her poetry children, house and home. Let us put beside Droste the most effective and the most widely read poetesses in the last century, the writers of elegant, unreally-pretty poetry and the general family novel reading. These are indeed in their emotional life genuine, lovable women and for that reason, in their literary achievements, entirely normal and conventional. But the great women achieved greatness—because they were great men.

Now Möbius, in the above-mentioned article, brings forward a second argument against women which has some connection with the question of genius. He says in fact : ' the period of intellectual bloom in most women is very short and extends at best into the early years of marriage. Thereafter a certain intellectual atrophy sets in which transforms the brilliant, spirited girl into a simple, comfortable, harmless woman.' " Whosoever has not had the chance to listen to the conversations of old women," said Möbius, " can hardly conceive the emptiness and wearisomeness of their chatter." At this point we must take the part of the women. Naturally the tea-time conversation of many old women belongs to the realm of weak-mindedness ; but what about the talk of old men at a drinking bar ?

Here we can derive important biological evidence from the students' song-book. It has often been lamented that students' songs only reflect four student years of life whilst the whole remaining term of life, the land of Philistia, is neglected as if it were a useless appendage, a mere yawning nothing. And yet in a certain sense the student songs are right. The average man as he grows older looks back with his philistine feelings on the time of his youth and says with involuntary conviction, ' I was a very different fellow then.' By that, he means a more valuable personality. This feeling is a very general one and it must have some biological basis. And in fact we see in the average man a greater freshness and animation of his whole intellectual attitude during the years of youth. Even in natures that later become most banal there are in youth a few attempts at independent thinking, the germ of some little musical, poetic or conversational talent, a little wit and spirit, all things which, in such averagely-gifted persons, slowly or suddenly disappear without trace after the twenty-fifth year. There remains little that one can call individuality after the demands of the working day, eating and sleeping have been met. And the dry-as-dust conventional occupations are not alone responsible, for the dust remains only where the ground is already inwardly dry. As soon as a tense personality arrives, even the driest of callings becomes full of spirit and life.

Thus " mutatio rerum," that familiar interjection which accompanies the students' song with its well-known melancholy lilt, is no sentimental phrase, but rather the expression of a deep biological revolution which is produced in the soul of the average man beyond puberty according to certain inner laws. True, the average man attains to the peak of his social usefulness, ripeness and experience, in middle age, but he reaches the climax of value in his personality, of independent intellectual creativeness, in the second half of adolescence. In the uncharitable and rather bombastic words of Möbius this truth would be expressed as follows :

After the twenty-fifth year there occurs in the average man a slight degree of permanent idiocy. In short, at this age begins not only the acquired physiological weak-mindedness of woman but also of man. The fundamental error of Möbius, however, consists in using everywhere as the measure of human worth a criterion derived from a relatively short interval in human life, the value of which is quite arbitrary.

Puberty has, in regard to the intellectual productivity of human beings, the effect of an intoxicating drug : this we call an hormone effect. Chemical changes in the blood, conditioned by the sexual ripening, act upon the brain like wine and bring out everything in the individual endowment and personality, even though it be only present in traces, to blossom and shine for a short time.

Such hormone effects, effects of the inner chemistry of living substances and especially of the stimulating juice of certain ductless glands, are to be found as essential factors not only in puberty but in every other kind of spiritual periodicity and phasic variation of life. Their power is so great that they can completely stunt and inhibit the expression of significant mental endowments even up to the second half of life and then suddenly let them spring forth magnificently with correspondingly greater vitality, finally perhaps to damp them down at the close of life. The spirit of genius too is no free-floating, absolute power, but is strictly bound to the laws of blood chemistry and the endocrine glands. One of the most remarkable examples of this is the life of the poet C. F. Meyer. He showed, in company with peculiar disturbance of skull growth and of the endocrine glands, a remarkable retardation of bodily development. Until his fortieth year he appeared stunted and as lean as a skeleton, and only at this age did his beard begin to grow and his figure to take on the later fullness and stateliness. And at this age for the first time appeared a collection of poems.

The mental differences of the sexes too, as far as they concern the problem of genius, rest essentially upon such hormone effects. It may be that these hormones produce certain mental dispositions similar in nature to the ' secondary sex characters '.

We have gone far into this connection because it is the starting-point for the whole understanding of periodic creativeness in the life of genius. We hear again the words of Goethe, ' Geniuses experience a second adolescence, whereas other people are only young once.' If we wish to get closer to the biological truth lying behind that statement we must first reject from our study the group of constitutional hypomanic persons, people like Goethe's mother and Field-marshal Blücher, on whose indestructible liveliness all ages of life roll by indifferently. Slight periodicity may indeed show itself in the most advanced old age, as with Blücher.

Quite apart from this group the life curve of highly gifted people shows a different form from that of normal people. After the storms of the actual period of adolescence, which by its especial boisterousness is more harmful than favourable to a balanced intellectual effort, there begins in these cases the most valuable part of the development of personality, precisely where it ceases in the average person. Then in a steady creative urge they produce their ripest and most individual works right on until the approach of old age. The summit of their lives comes where one falsely supposes it to come for all men, at the prime of life. At that time they lose none of their youthful freshness,

I

spirituality and breadth, indeed they gain from the clearing up of their emotional impulses. Even the approaching stiffening of old age only serves to make the firm outlines of their personalities still more imposing. This type of life curve among men of genius ; disturbing violence and storminess at puberty, followed by a steady productiveness rising to the prime of life, we find clearly exemplified in Schiller for the first part of his life and for the whole course of life in Bismarck.

We can point to the Schiller-Bismarck form of intellectual development as the fundamental type of life curve in genius. But if the creative urge of genius is dominated not by a uniformly - working disposition but a variety of changing biological influences, there arise very varied and quite paradoxical pictures. Of these the regular cyclic wave curve, as in the case of Goethe, is most closely related to normal psychological development. But quite bizarre is the nature of the circular-paranoiac type, as seen in Robert Mayer, where a person, suddenly, in the middle of his life, becomes fired with genius, brings forth a single great conception and then for the rest of his life sinks down again into the ranks of average mentalities.

An astonishing, though fairly frequent and typical life curve, is that found in such men as Ludwig Uhland or Scheffel. These men brought forth in adolescence, or shortly after adolescence, a single masterpiece, Scheffel producing *Ekkehard* and Uhland his lyrics and ballads. Then suddenly, just when one is expecting the richest blossoms, genius is gone, perhaps without leaving a trace behind, and never comes again. Such men may nevertheless be always somewhat more intellectual and richer in personality throughout their remaining days than is the average man, but compared with the meteoric brilliance of their youth they are severely stunted. These cases stand within the realm of schizophrenic mental disturbance or dementia praecox. They set forth the normal life curve in an exaggerated, even caricatured, form, in that the upward swing at puberty is more striking and the downward gradient thereafter steeper than is usually the case. Here we find all transition forms between the normal development of ' physiological weak-mindedness ' and severe typical cases of dementia praecox. With Uhland the relapse from adolescence followed a healthy course, barely perceptible as a certain drying-up of the springs of artistic vitality. In Scheffel there were slight, repeated attacks of mental disturbance, with acute depressions and delusions of persecution. Finally in Hölderlin we encounter the fully developed drama of severe schizophrenic collapse, which leaves behind for all the years of manhood and old age a spiritual ruin.

A converse phenomenon is the abnormal retardation of the onset of puberty. The poet C. F. Meyer presents us with an uncommon case which would be exceptional even in the realm of psychiatry. Here a paradoxical functioning of the endocrine glands turned the whole course of his development topsy-turvy, for his youth was the deepest winter of his life and spring came to him only in the later years of manhood. A similar life curve exists to some extent in Dostoievsky and Liliencron. One of the most personal notes in his poems and one which no other poet can relive, is this unprecedented late awakening of the soul in the afternoon of his life ; this desire to enjoy in a few swift minutes the flowing stream of happiness and vitality in a youth which is almost past. Like one awakening from some evil stupor he now writes :

> " I was as one bound by a heavy spell ;
> Life had not reached me : I lay stiffly in dream.
> And now a thousand unused hours
> Swirl boisterously around me."

But now the spring awoke in him something different from the sense of life's sorrow which the young poet usually produces in himself. It awoke a more bitter, personal experience.

> " The heart that has missed its youthful days
> Is damned to wander forth,
> When the spring sun flames again
> And the wave breaks into foam.
>
> Oh, the pain of forfeited youth !
> The heart seeks ever for its springtime,
> Seeks for it as for lost treasure,
> Gone for ever, gone for ever."

If C. F. Meyer had died with his fortieth year the few people who knew him might have stood at his grave-side shrugging their shoulders, half pitiful, half relieved. They would have thought of him as an ungifted, rather eccentric son of a highly respected family. In Zürich they might have called him the cross and shame of his family, a failure, an ill-spent existence. In order to do everything possible for him they had placed his very talentless poetry before the poet Gustav Pfizer, but he had felt quite unable to encourage him in that line. His younger sister was forced at length to learn some profession because her twenty-eight-year-old brother earned nothing and was a burden on the family means. His mother considered it a great step forward when her son, long grown to manhood, took leave of the muses, but then she was forced to dissuade him from thoughts of marriage. At one time she wrote about him : " My poor son remains always in practically the same condition. He retains his melancholy disposition and his incorrigible incapacity to take up any regular work. He suffers much from his inability to aim at any goal or take up any career, or in any way make up his mind. He manages to fill up his time with reading, a few studies and lonely walks, but these things do not seem to improve his position in any way. I too am compelled to admit that I have come to expect nothing more of him in this world."

Shy of human beings, dejected, wrapped in dreams and bitterly confined within himself, he wandered here and there, tried this and that, all to no avail. He wanted to be a painter, then a poet and a lawyer, but nowhere did he show real talent. He tried making translations, gave lessons and began to study again himself. At one time he travelled to Paris and Berlin, dreamed away his time and returned to Zürich, read insatiably and to no real purpose and on one occasion actually wished to busy himself with a history of the Apostles. Friends of the family had to look after him and his mother was much concerned to provide the cost of his living. He had a big, lonely garden in which he used to walk alone, always threading the same snake-like path around the lawns, disappearing deep within the shrubbery and taking to flight instantly if he unexpectedly encountered anyone. In the end people took him for dead, for he never showed himself and only went out at night on lonely wanderings through the empty streets.

His manner acquired a sharp, irritable quality. Even in times of momentary happiness he would be suddenly seized by an acute nervous anxiety ; he would burst into tears and be unable to answer any questions. Or he would suddenly break out with sharp wounding words, so that the relations with his tender, sensitive mother became temporarily intolerable. He disliked having any bodily contact with people and when anyone greeted him he would offer only two fingers of the right hand.

He went to a lunatic asylum for the first time in his twenty-seventh year. There he suffered from melancholy, hypochondria and insane delusions in which he believed, for example, that all people found him disgusting and afflicted with noisome breath. " The feeling took hold of him," said a friend, " that he lived in the midst of emptiness. He had actually no real contact with life but floated about in the web of his own brain, having no duties, no social life and no order in his daily life. He despaired of himself and came near to making a deliberate end to his life." That also is a note in his poems that one is bound to recognise. Once, whilst making a lonely cruise, he swam out into the lake until he had quite lost sight of his boat and it was nearly midnight before he returned home. A dark spirit called to him out of the gloomy waste of waters as with the voice of his mother ; his mother, who, in the midst of profound melancholy, had made an end of herself by jumping into the lake. " A dear, dear voice called to me constantly out of the watery abyss." And in the rushes along the shore he saw pale, whispering ghosts that waved to him. Or he heard the merry laughter of dead friends rising out of the waves in the dead of night.

And now, as he approached his fortieth year, these unreal, ghostly urges suddenly came to an end and he celebrated the transformation in song as the breaking of blessed dawn into a darkened cell. From his thirty-ninth to his sixty-seventh year C. F. Meyer produced the whole of his art. True, he suffered even in later life from the over-sensitiveness of his nerves, from moody fluctuations of feeling and sudden lassitude. Beneath an outward appearance of stolidity and calm he had a highly sensitive, emotional life, which was readily wounded even by the most remote discords and which found violent emotion, either in himself or in others, quite intolerable. Yet however lonely, however shy of reality and lacking in sensory joys his life may have been, it was still a life that was worth the living. It bore the richest fruit and was ever and anon lit up by some solitary ecstasy of happiness which threw a great, calm, golden glow over the declining afternoon of his existence.

EIGHTH CHAPTER

The Scientist

" GENIUS is the capacity for taking pains " a famous
writer has said. If we are to suppose that he intended
anything but a witticism thereby, we must strenuously
contradict him. The Greeks had practically the opposite
notion in that they expected genius to show the greatest
possible detachment from regular labour. Their view that
monotonous, daily work for one's living was dangerous to
intellectual originality, that it made it banausic, has a kernel
of truth. Naturally, one must admit that the Greek method
of preserving intellectual power is only possible in the childhood of civilisation where one may produce new intellectual
values without having to acquire skill and without troubling
to acquaint oneself with a great deal of accumulated knowledge. Science, certainly, is no longer essentially served by
witty discourses but only by industrious research and intelligent application to professional work.

And yet industry alone will not produce anything new
even in science, still less will it produce anything resembling
the work of scientific genius. We are fond of characterising
science in contradistinction to art as ' dry ' and imagining
to ourselves that scientific systems are produced as by a
thousand assiduous bees uniformly setting cell upon cell.
In reality the progress of science takes place largely according
to the formula of Schiller, *i.e.* through a few master architects,
or in any case through a number of guiding brains which

constantly set all the industrious labourers at work for decades. Actual research work, however, is no more dry than the activities of a great poet or prophet. Like these it is frequently controlled by a spirit, by strong passions and sudden intuitions. And as such it is the product of quite definite mechanisms of thought and feeling, bound by psychological laws to certain mental endowments which relatively few people possess.

There are many great investigations which, at least when viewed from afar, seem to have been carried out with calm, lucid matter-of-factness. Whether it is possible to complete a great investigation solely by immense intellectual power and cool detachment is a question which can at present be entertained but not answered. One can certainly not answer it in the affirmative. Most of the biographical material dealing with great scientists is signally lacking in psychological insight. Of course there may have been many great men of learning whose natures were entirely stolid and uninteresting. But there is clear psychological evidence that the most significant scientists, who have produced great conceptions, have frequently shown a very lively originality and vibrated with sensibility and inward tension. Behind the cool stream of thought there lies a glowing passionate core and sometimes, carefully guarded, an autistic world of desires. There are classical cases in which some great deprivation, some heavy blow from life, has turned a man into scientific work and been the starting-point of greater scientific achievements. In these cases calm detachment has not been the primary possession of that personality, but has been attained by a fanatical struggle, and can only be regarded as the steely end-product of an immense inner struggle.

Scientific research, in so far as it is the work of genius, is to be explained largely according to the psychiatric formula of ' overvaluation ', or, as one used to say, of the ' fixed idea.' Men of strong reasoning powers, who are nevertheless possessed of a fixed idea, are characterised so far as they are abnormal, by the term paranoiac. The paranoiac thinker is usually a man of tenacious and deep emotionality who, through some acute experience, is forced into a definite line of thought. He then pursues the line of thought relentlessly and with the greatest consistency, so that his spiritual life becomes more and more tyrannically and one-sidedly controlled by it. With the fixation of such an overvalued idea in the emotional life of the individual there generally enters a systematised delusion, *i.e.* an increased power of combining impressions, extending even to the smallest and most negligible matters of daily life, into a support for the original belief. Ultimately the controlling system of thought develops a whole array of tributary ideas, whilst everything that is of no use to it is shut out of consciousness and overlooked with complete, passionate blindness. Such overvalued ideas arise every day in connection with passionate love and party politics. They can bring those who entertain them into the deepest misfortune or the lunatic asylum, or drive them to the greatest deeds, according to the favourableness of circumstances and the intellectual power of the individual. But they are always great forces in the soul.

It is generally unusual passions that bring forth unusual ideas. When the feelings are allowed to run free and the paths of thought are loosened, then the unusual will arise and bring genius, perversions or madness, according to circumstances. With many great scientists and inventors passionate emotions develop which drive their thought constantly in the same direction, producing the utmost tension, until at last a short circuit occurs : somewhere a spark leaps to a new spot where up till then no human thought has ever passed. Then the old and established ways of thought are destroyed. Thus arise new ideas and discoveries. Genius *is* industry—of course. But not the simple capacity for taking pains. Not extensive, but intensive industry ; industry that is directed with unbalanced ardour upon a definite point. Scientific and inventive genius is industry under the sway of an overvalued idea.

Think of Count Zeppelin who for years lost one airship after another over the Bodensee. With unswerving tenacity he spent all his means in the service of this idea of the dirigible airship, an idea which all normally-constituted citizens had already recognised as premature and impossible. At that time people were inclined to regard Count Zeppelin as a poor, harmless fool who ought properly to be cared for in an asylum. But in the moment that success came to him he was transformed from a nominally, mentally-diseased paranoiac to " the most famous man of the twentieth century."

Did this success change his personality in any way ? Was he in no way a genius before when he continued, with this blind ' delusion of invention ' in his head, to waste his means and ruin his reputation ? Or, if he was a fool before, did he become less of a fool because everybody had praised him as a genius ?

There are successful and unsuccessful inventors. The unsuccessful ones are called paranoiacs.

Through the overvalued idea there arises very obviously in certain scientists and inventors a narrowing of the field of mental vision which results frequently in a positively

grotesque neglect of everyday life. Absent-mindedness is a
proverbial characteristic of learned men. Perhaps one ought
to say : ' Overconcentration of attention,' which leaves the
individual blind and deaf to all else. It is a kind of auto-
hypnosis, a strained staring at a single point. The ability
to gather the whole mental energy into a single focus is a
characteristic associative peculiarity of many scientists,
which, of course, is derived largely from the inherited dispositions and cannot be acquired by training.

Again, the urge to bring the most trivial happenings of
daily life into relation with the overvalued idea, which in
paranoiacs we call the delusional tendency, is found frequently
among scientists of genius. It has often been some insignificant, everyday experience encountered by discoverers who
have for years penetrated in one direction of thought with
single-minded passion, that has caused the final short circuit,
the last leaping spark of genius. Such an occurrence is
related of Galileo who, perceiving the swinging lamp in the
cathedral, formulated the law of oscillation of pendulums.

The discovery of the law of the conservation of energy
by the Heilbronn medical doctor, Robert Mayer, followed a
similar course. This man, extremely passionate and temperamental from his earliest years, was already outstanding
in his student days on account of the originality of his
thought, which expressed itself now in effervescent wit and
now in some astonishing leap of ideas. He was also notorious
for his constant absent-mindedness. Disturbances of associa-
tion were also very prominent with him : it was almost
impossible in conversation to hold him to any train of
thought ; he would leap rapidly to the ultimate conclusions,
leaving out all the intermediate terms. No sooner had his
lively wit endeared him to a social circle than his abruptness

would estrange everybody, for in conversation he paid no heed to the appropriateness of his remarks to the topic under discussion. Moreover, this peculiar thinking apparatus was driven by such a powerful temperament that his mentality knew no bounds either in friendly approaches or on his outbursts of rage, which would last sometimes for days.

Already as a ten-year-old boy the sight of a mill at work brought him to the question of the conservation and transformation of energy, in connection with the related problem of perpetual motion. He worried at this one idea and it began more and more to take full possession of his mind. On an ocean voyage in his twenty-sixth year, which he had undertaken as ship's doctor on the way to the Dutch Indies, he was led by a couple of chance observations to the decisive ideas which set his mind on fire. One was the observation of the steersman that after storms the sea was warmer than before. Then, in the docks at Surabaya, he was called upon to bleed a sailor and he noticed that the venous blood here, in the tropics, was not dark red, as in cooler zones, but bright red. With one of those sudden leaps of thought which were so characteristic, he derived from this fact of biological heat regulation the law of the mechanical equivalent of heat.

That glance at the bright red blood of the sailor had so impressed him that in the following weeks he forgot to write up his diary and, full of this one idea, took the next ship back home. On the way home, after suffering from rapid changes of mood between gaiety and misery, he broke out in violent ' deliria ', attacks of sudden excitement and mental disturbance which lasted for days.

After he had returned home, got married and started as a practising doctor in Heilbronn, he set himself forthwith to the expression of his ideas in writing. These appeared at three-year intervals in the four communications : " Observations on the forces of inorganic nature," 1842 ; " Organic movement and its connection with metabolism," 1845 ; "A contribution to celestial dynamics," 1848, and finally the comprehensive work, fitting all together : " Observations on the mechanical equivalent of heat," 1851.

Mayer's wife has recorded that during this decisive period of his life all the neighbourhood was struck by his extraordinary mental condition, especially by his tendency to sudden, immoderate states of excitement. There were also—she expresses it almost tenderly—' moments when he was rather unreasonable,' in which he broke up the furniture and tore his clothes to pieces. Of his immediate neighbours, mainly his wife, he made weird, impossible and unreasonable demands. He was, as he himself admits, thoroughly childish at times.

In the years following his Indian voyage of 1840 Mayer became so entirely engrossed in thinking out the problems and consequences of his theories that it became very difficult even in ordinary conversation to talk to him about anything else. So far did this go that he acquired the habit of greeting and taking leave of his friends in scientific maxims, as ' causa aequat effectum ', ' ex nihilo nihil fit ' and ' nihil fit ad nihilum.'

Scarcely had Robert Mayer commenced the publication of his works when a battle began in the scientific world to decide, firstly, whether the law of conservation of energy might be true, and, secondly, whether Robert Mayer could claim to be its originator. To begin with, the world of learned societies scarcely paid any attention to the work of this unknown medical practitioner, who was for them an outsider. The famous Helmholtz treated him for years with cursory scorn, and Seyffer, in the *Augsburger Allgemeinen Zeitung*, had ever for him only a number of unsparing and insulting observations. Mayer, intoxicated with the greatness of his idea, had promised himself that his writings would bring him fame and cause a sensation in the scientific world. Now he was thrown into the most restless moodiness by strained hopes and severely disappointed expectations, pitchforked for years from momentary states of pride to equally passing depressions of his self-esteem. In energetic polemics written to the Paris Academy of Science he defended his fame as a discoverer against the English physicist Joule, who believed himself to have discovered the law.

The excitement of the struggle reached its climax in the early part of 1850 with the controversial publication of Seyffer, by which Mayer felt himself to be personally insulted. He tried by letters to the *Allgemeinen Zeitung* and personal appeals to the editor to get a hearing, but in vain. Mayer did not possess the capacity of most men to get rid of an evil emotional incubus by seeking diversion. Instead he persisted in the same obstinate line of thought, turning neither to the right nor to the left. Just as, previously, it had always been impossible for him to leave the scientific ideas with which he had been busied, now it was impossible for him to get out of his head the injustice that he had suffered in their service. He was utterly enraged by his treatment at the hands of the press and scientific societies ; the consolations of his friends were fruitless, he could write nothing more and spent his nights without gaining any rest or refreshment.

Finally on a hot, close night in spring, which he had spent restlessly tossing on his bed, he was seized by a violent attack of madness. Clothed only in his night attire he sprang, before the eyes of his instantly awakened wife, out of a second floor window on to the asphalt street beneath, where he lay severely injured.

His spiritual convalescence did not proceed parallel to his physical recovery. Already in the last years of the struggle over his discovery, somewhat before 1850, Mayer had manifested a peculiar turn toward a strict religiosity, founded on a literal interpretation of the Bible. The cold causality of the law of energy which he had discovered, destructive of all mysticism, stood in grotesque opposition to this new system of beliefs, and he himself occasionally became aware of the strange contradiction. Certainly the bitter disappointments of his career as a scientist had much to do with this sudden swing of his intellectual interests from the scientifically exact to the mystically religious, though doubtless the ultimate cause lay still deeper and is only to be understood from psychiatry.

Robert Mayer himself asserted : " It is possible that the continued suspension of any recognition of my work, upon which I had counted so much, was the fundamental reason for the temporary cooling-off of my scientific ardour. It is certain that my interest in transcendental religious truths came upon me with irresistible power at that time. The power to concentrate exclusively on one thing, and all the passionate hastiness which I, as a very temperamental man, have to confess to, were transferred at once to this new realm. I must now acknowledge without reserve what at that time I had firmly forbidden myself to think about. There lived in me a desire for recognition, and however much I might strive to thrust down this feeling as one of sinful pride it was beyond my power to do so. I could not stifle my scientific consciousness, and the systematic opposition which everywhere faced my assertions was bound to call forth a bitterness which rose in me from day to day." This struggle which Mayer describes, between the embittered, tense feelings of the scientist and the despondent, self-accusatory religious ideas of sin, which split up his spiritual life during the second half of his labour of genius, must be seized upon as the key to a deeper psychiatric understanding of the whole course of his creative genius. The ' interphase ' in manic-depressive afflictions, with its tense mixture of feelings such as we see here, and its tendency to produce ' paranoiac ', overvalued ideas, has already been carefully, scientifically studied. But the pathological drive in Mayer's religious conversion had, even at that time, struck one of his contemporaries, who wrote : " Even in the way in which Mayer embraced this positive religious standpoint there lay a certain restless anxiety and lack of balance."

Therewith a longer mental disturbance set in which lasted until the autumn of 1853—two years altogether. The psychosis consisted of a periodic coming and going, at intervals of several days, of violent maniacal outbursts. The intervals between the outbursts would begin with melancholic depression and conviction of sin. Later they were occupied by gay moods of a manic type in which Robert Mayer would give himself up to unbridled merriment and general observations highly pleasing to himself.

The second section of Robert Mayer's life is, still more than the first, characterised by regular recurring, abnormal fluctuations of emotion. Naturally the excitement never again attained the strength of the 1852 outbursts, yet on three later occasions Mayer was compelled to stay in the sanatorium at Kennenburg for some months. That was in

K

1856, 1865 and 1871. Yet outside the asylum his periods of excitement were characterised by the greatest destructiveness, by amazing spite against those around him and by violent outbursts of rage lasting hours, days and nights, during which he constantly rushed about the house and drank heavily of spiritous liquors. Towards the end of these outbursts there usually came a depressed, melancholic mood and a tendency to reproach himself. In between times he continued to carry on his medical practice, though to a limited extent.

From 1851 to 1862 he disappeared from the scientific world without trace. He wrote absolutely nothing and his admirers told themselves that he was benighted in incurable madness or had died in a lunatic asylum. Only after 1862 did Robert Mayer begin to be a famous man ; that was after the leading English physicist, Tyndall, had fought for the recognition of his services to science with such personal warmth.

One may add that with growing age the periods of excitement became milder and more rare. Robert Mayer died on the 20th March 1878, heaped with the honours which came to him in the evening of his life from all corners of Europe.

Robert Mayer's career as an investigator is a strange one. Suddenly on a sea voyage, in the incipient stages of an acute manic psychosis, he feels illuminated by this idea of a law of physical energy, as by a flash of lightning. He drops everything, leaves his regular written diary from that day, walks about absent-mindedly for years, is incapable of any ordinary conversation, employs Latin formulae from physics for greetings, behaves like a naughty child, destroys furniture and clothes, writes, in spite of all, four immortal treatises, and struggles, laughed at by the professional world, to the Parisian Academy itself. He fights for his system in all the learned bodies of Europe, and ends up as a raving maniac in an asylum. And two years later, when he is better, he becomes a normal citizen and doctor, who for eleven years never takes a pen in his hand again.

Compared with the violent pulse of Robert Mayer's temperament the beating waves of Goethe's life make a gently-swinging idyll. Robert Mayer was no academic authority, but an enthusiastic lunatic, a person possessed, a priest of Bacchus—hunted across the sea by an idea, hurled out of a window, raving with wrath and inspiration. And between the two high peaks of excitement in his middle life, product of a few tense years, appears his one great idea—one of the great ideas of a century of natural science. Out of the mad whirl of a psychosis it rose, lighting up everything like a rocket for a few all-too-bright moments. Before that he was quite unknown, after, for the rest of his life, he was intellectually dead, a person in whom every spark of genius had been extinguished.

NINTH CHAPTER

Heroes and Leaders

BISMARCK lives in the general consciousness as the figure of an old Teutonic knight, a right valiant old soldier ; emitting a stream of power and vigour. He is thought of as the smith of empire with the athletic muscles and the will of steel, as the man of blood and iron, who feared God, but nothing else in the world. In short, he is conceived as the prototype of unbroken strength, sanity and German stalwartness.

In reality Bismarck appeared quite different. The English painter Richmond said of him : " He is altogether a most attractive, amiable and sensitive person, a thoroughly fine gentleman. I asked him if he could really be the iron Bismarck. ' No,' he replied, ' my hardness is entirely artificial. I am all nerves and to such an extent that self-control has been the hardest lesson of my life '." That this was no idle phrase, will be evident from the facts. Bismarck, the grandson of a delicate, highly-strung invalid and the son of a mother who was in a constantly delicate state, whose restless irritability, lack of real emotion and hard egoism stamps her as a degenerate, hysteric type. Bismarck's youth and especially his adolescent development is charac-terised in the highest degree by restless dissatisfaction and a lack of spiritual steadiness or equilibrium. From his student days to the time of his engagement he was impelled by mad, ill-balanced urges to outdo all others in wild drinking bouts, riding and affairs of honour. The origin of these impulses is not found in an untamed joy of youth but in a dark moodiness and a complete antagonism to God and all the world. Hence his characteristic failure to choose a profession, his oscillation between the career of an estate owner and a government official, which seemed never likely to solve itself, and all his impulsive, emotional actions, exemplified by the occasion when he suddenly disappeared without leave on account of a temporary infatuation. His moods leapt restlessly between the utmost extremes, between heavy sentimental emotionality, and the cold elegance of the man of the world, between complete sceptical atheism and strictly orthodox religious pietism. His explosive, impulsive irritability is well known through the beautiful anecdote in which the young Bismarck, enraged through being kept waiting in the anteroom by President von Meding, gave orders to the hall-porter : " Tell His Excellency the President that I have gone away and that I shall not be coming back again."

In the prime of his life, too, Bismarck was never a man of steady and calmly collected power. His nervous excitability was as much feared by those working with him as his eccentric mode of life, which turned night into day, for he would dictate feverishly all the night long and then sleep on until well past midday. What a droll comparison is there between 'the poor, sick duck,' as Bismarck was occasionally called by his wife, and the steely Germanic knight who appears in the popular conception. His wife knew him for the man he was, upset on every occasion by nervous excitement, a prey to colds and rheumatism and constantly ill in bed with nerve pains ; a man who, at the great moments of history, as at the battle of Königgratz, was overcome with nervous fits of weeping, and who lay abed and vomited gall when he had been severely annoyed.

Can then Bismarck still be considered the stalwart old veteran ? Certainly ! But at the same time, is he not much more to be regarded as the most artful old fox in the inveterate game of intrigue to which European diplomacy had degenerated ? Was he not an unscrupulous national egoist, a player who played dangerously with the royal throne and the existence of the state as his last desperate stakes, a cold, calculating man who stirred up a revolution in Hungary whilst remaining the most morose reactionary in his own land ; a man who met Napoleon's cunning with greater cunning and used him to his own ends, and a man who would be a Conservative to-day out of the profound sanction of his emotions and a Liberal to-morrow for tactical reasons ? And when we look at Bismarck again as a representative of his country in foreign lands we find him a spoilt, pretentious, drawing-room man, who found French manners too coarse and could only tolerate the cream of Russian aristocracy in social intercourse. Here he is the courtier, over-civilised to the point of decadence, the elegant conversationalist, the close friend of the Queen Mother, the gentleman who waxed eloquent over Beethoven sonatas with Russian countesses in the moonlight. At one and the same period we see him as a being whom music moved to tears, a lonely, dreaming lover of nature, a tender, attentive husband and a clever stylist, a man of political witticisms and of finely turned oratorical points. The more one delves into the personality of Bismarck the more one discovers him to be complex, modern, highly strung and changing from day to day.

It is true that Bismarck was also upright, true, courageous

and a good deal more. He was the highly complicated, yet predictable result of an inheritance in which the simple, unshakable power of the paternal family of landed gentry had become mixed, in an almost impossible contrast, with the highly-strung, incipiently decadent, but highly-gifted mentality of the maternal family from the intelligentsia. Without these nervous tensions and bizarre contrasts of character within him he would probably have remained a coarse-fibred, capable, country squire, as all his forefathers had been for centuries. It was only the nervous irritability and psychopathic lack of balance in his mother's family which had brought this impulsive urgency to great deeds into the more stolid paternal stock. For great actions never spring from healthy, satisfied states but only from inner turmoil and restlessness. He who becomes a genius does so only because he is forced, because inner tensions are driving him constantly to new output. The father's inheritance of vigorous, primitive force was of no more value for the tasks of modern life than the uncouth weapon of a giant, but the tortuous intellect and the almost decadent over-refinement of feeling which came to him from his city-bred mother, enabled him to use that power through labyrinths of intrigue, and again, it was that highly-strung, psychopathic restlessness which alone urged him into the fray at all.

This is the true picture of Bismarck : the warrior figure of an old Hun with the brain of a modern neurasthenic, the most thick-headed country squire and the most enlightened man of the world in one breath, an inconceivable mixture of elegance, brutality, civilisation and primitive emotional depth, of massive stolidity and perverse irritability, a spoilt intellectual with the tough instincts of a peasant, a genius, whose will-power is goaded by the weakness of his nerves.

Courage among heroes of early times, before man became a domesticated animal, meant primitive combativeness, born of constant, bitter need. At that time too, fighting came to be in peaceful times one of the few possible ways in which a man could exercise his physical energy and satisfy the need of his soul for excitement and activity. Above all it enabled him to satisfy the predatory animal's lust for blood, for destruction and the cruel infliction of pain ; a lust which even to-day, hidden in the heroic gestures of military leaders, seeks to smash with one blow of its claw all the fine products of the civilisation which is trying to tame it. The heroes of the old sagas and folk stories, who rushed forward with Homeric cries, rending shield and helmet, were in reality somewhat like the present-day peasant youths of, *e.g.* Upper Bavaria, who consider that a church consecration without a knife fight is no proper ceremony. Deeds which in primitive times helped one to immortality now sink to the level of illegal breaches of the peace. In the broad light of modern civilised society the bold adventurer is but a vagabond, and the cunning Ulysses can only count now, as with Captain von Köpenick, on a most modest literary glorification. Generally, in times of peaceful, civilised development, poets and thinkers stand higher in public esteem than warriors, because they create new and productive values in civilisation. But in early times the thinker developed in the shadow of the man of action ; the priest, the bard, the leech and the artistic smith were significant but subsidiary figures besides the cult of the hero. Thereafter, as the still, high summer days of human history approached, the discoverer, the man of brain, the scientist and the artist became honoured with the name of genius ; indeed the conception of genius has developed with them historically.

But as soon as a great calamity breaks over civilised people, the man of action enters into his birthright. Yet he is now no longer an elementary being, even courage and will-power have become complex moral exercises. Power alone is entirely worthless here ; only through refined sensitiveness and intellectual deliberation can the hero of a great civilised people thread his way through the complex battlefield of modern life. For that reason the greatest heroes of modern times have had in them a good deal of the man of brain, of the artist, the literary and scientific man. Frederick the Great, according to his intellectual interests, was at least as much a philosopher, historian and fine man of letters as he was statesman and general. Moltke, as is well known, began his career with novel writing. He was rightly called the philosopher of battles, and his fine, intellectual head, the head of a man of learning, was far different from that of a simple Homeric hero. And Bismarck, one of the cleverest stylists that the German language has known, had to thank for the effective half of his inheritance the learned family on his mother's side. Naturally it is of advantage to the personality of a modern leader if he has retained through a series of civilised ancestors a good part of the root instincts of elementary boldness, pugnacity and toughness, the virtues of the old warrior knights. The personalities which remind one most of the figures of early times are those hypomanic, pushful individuals, like old Blücher. He belonged to the men who only feel happy when they are in a fight and who, like the old Germans, can summon up nothing but contempt for prolonged contemplativeness and idle musing. Service in a garrison he called ' martyrdom in idleness '. Without constantly renewed risk, life had no charm for him, and in quiet times of peace he sought stimulus for his love of daring in playing for high stakes at games of chance. To such games he was as passionately devoted as were the old Viking warriors, and indeed he lost large sums of money in this way. His skill as a general was more akin to the swift, audacious tactics of the hussar than to cleverly-thought-out, artistic strategy, and the way in which he managed men was entirely instinctive, direct and homely.

In his way Blücher had an original and very buoyant mentality but lacked a comprehensive intellect. And like many simple heroic natures, Blücher, as a general, received a uniform estimate from friend and foe alike. Most great men of action since classical times, *e.g.* in Germany, Wallenstein, Frederick the Great and Bismarck, or Caesar and Napoleon, impress one as highly complex and problematic characters beside Blücher. They are certainly men of the strangest inner contradictions of character, extending to the moral realm. Their courage and will-power is not something elementary but the result of complicated and varied psychological mechanisms. The favourite figure in the phantasies of modern literature, the so-called ' 100-per-cent.-man ', has never existed in reality. As the superman he was an invention of Friedrich Nietzsche, a speculative, historical construction, compounded on the one side from the ' blond beast ', the robust, primitive, berserk hero, and on the other from the perverted, decadent intriguers, despots and poisoners among the princes of the Italian Renaissance. It is thus a strange mixture of Florence and the Teutoburger Forest, of *Waltharilied* and Machiavelli. Here the beginning and the end of biological development, a figure out of the childhood of the race, and a product of over-ripeness in highly developed periods of civilisation, are thrust forcibly together, and the

result is held up as the ' superman ' for an ideal of the future
to guide human evolution. Nietzsche's hero was supposed
to combine the utmost health and sanity with the highest
genius. Such a combination does not exist. It is a magnificent, stimulating, ideal conception, but, unfortunately, a
biological absurdity. The superman in this form, as the goal
of human breeding, is about as attainable as the ideal horse
projected by a stud farm which attempted to breed a
thoroughbred race-horse that one could use at the same
time for heavy labour like a wild, weather-beaten horse of
the steppe.

So it is also with the ' will to power ' which some imagine
constitutes the one fundamental instinct in the genius of
action. Many who have the will to power fail in spite of
all striving to play any effective part in history, whilst
hesitating, shy, meditating men, who advance slowly and
irresolutely, constantly stepping back from the decisive act,
become in spite of themselves a sure pillar in great national
catastrophes, when once the passions of the crowd have
closed around them. An example is at hand in the German
Renaissance, where Ulrich von Hutten strove for the reins of
intellectual and political leadership, whilst they were thrust
with much resistance into the hands of Martin Luther.
Such men as Luther, who become leaders and popular heroes
despite their inveterate pondering and self-criticism, can in
no way be explained by the psychological formula of the
will to power. Luther had first to pull himself through
periods of profound depression and the only struggle he ever
really fought was with the dark powers of his own soul.
Like Schiller, he was blindly swung on the wheel of time.
Circumstances threw him into opposition with the Pope.
Then the hostility to the harsh father of his childhood years,

like a thorn in his heart, urging him to revolutionary behaviour, expressed itself in adult life, by his attacking the father image in the form of the Pope, and with the weapons of learning. Then he is pressed forward against his will, step by step, by the inevitable course of events, as was the astrologising Wallenstein, to-day pushing one step onward, to-morrow drawing two steps backward. He is lifted on the shields of furious peasants, played with as a pawn by shrewd princes, grimly laughing and raging with inner uncertainty, with the storm wind of the times in his sails, tugging fearfully at all the old mooring-ropes—the hero and the explosive power of his century—and yet not a will to power, but a power in spite of will.

In connection with the Nietzschean system of ideas, Adler has given a general demonstration of " the unconditional primacy of the Will to Power, a leading fiction, which sets in more violently, more prematurely, and becomes more hastily completed, the more acutely the child's actual organic inferiority is allowed to bring his inferiority feeling into the foreground." He has brought some clear formulae and convincing observations, largely out of neurotic psychology, to demonstrate this point. We are taught that the gestures of the ' strong man ' are but the tricks of self-assurance, the protective mimicry of one essentially weak ; that striving for power is but an overcompensation for a feeling of inferiority. From the fine oratorical career of the stutterer Demosthenes down to the present day, there are innumerable examples of overcompensation in the history of famous men. And yet one must object that the neglect of inherited factors in this, as in all systems of predominantly environmental psychology, must lead to false conclusions. One cannot reduce the individual and all his character properties to a series of camouflages, adopted according to his position in the battle of life. Somewhere behind the scenes must be a point from which the stage properties are thrust forth and moved. There alone shall we find the primary self, *i.e.* the sum of inherited dispositions and capacities of reaction. And these must be regarded as varying extensively from one individual to another, however much the school of Adler may wish to overlook the fact. It is impossible to solve all problems of personality on this one theme of overcompensated inferiority feeling, without cheapening and misusing a theory which, in its proper place, and aptly applied, can yield good results. The problem of the exceptional performances of genius is not to be exhausted by this simple psychiatric formula, because it is never possible to ignore the factor of special intellectual talents in the inherited disposition. Thousands of nervous people needing assurance in life overcompensate their weaknesses, yet with all their striving they arrive at nothing but neuroses, empty theatricality, or a hard-gained display of average talent. Only a minority come to socially valuable exploits by this path, and very rarely, through favourable inheritance, does an exceptional case reach genius through the spasmodic tensions of neurosis.

Besides, overcompensation does not appear in all people of weak vitality. In clinical practice one meets many more people of weak nervous dispositions who have settled into a persistent, asthenic, weary, depressed and despondent attitude to life without making any serious attempt to derive therefrom a positive position of power. Overcompensation arises rather where there are, beside the asthenic components in the primary disposition, genuine factors of positive self-assertion and desire for power. These contrasting parts of the disposition, then take up opposite poles within the personality and produce a sharp mutual tension and repulsion. If now the sthenic components are sufficiently strong they may become overstimulated by the reaction of the accompanying asthenic traits and so be driven to the most extreme feats of power. This sthenic-asthenic polarity is, as we have already seen, a dynamic factor of the first rank not only in the realm of psychiatry, as a cause of insanity, but also in the great creations of men of genius.

Thus one notices at once in Luther the sharpest feelings of insufficiency, depression, fear, torturing uncertainty of mind and a clinging to definite, traditional symbols, which have all the characters of a compulsion neurosis. But side by side with these, one finds symptoms of rough, peasant vitality, of force and drive in verbal expression, triumphant humour, firmness in personal danger and a purely physically impressive tempo in the vigour of his literary productions. Similarly there stands in Bismarck, beside the abnormal susceptibility to excitement and general vulnerability of the vegetative nervous system, a rude health of the most important bodily organs which enabled him to attain a ripe old age in spite of his pernicious modes of life and the great hardships which he had earlier endured. Naturally the sthenic elements of one's make-up need not lie in such extraneous physical qualities ; they may equally well be present as tenacity of will, reasoning power, schizoid autism or hypomanic factors of constitution. The greatest feats of spiritual power therefore, do not arise out of simple power, still less out of the neurotic's mimicry of power, but rather from the tensions of inner, sthenic-asthenic polarity. In numerous cases this polarity is derived, as with Bismarck, from a great dissimilarity of the maternal and paternal inheritances, *i.e.* through ' germinal hostility '.

Yet there are forms of heroic leadership quite different from these. They are founded upon frigidity of temperament, indifference to hardship and danger, pedantic tenacity and autistic blindness to difficulties in the realisation of desired ideological systems. This typical symptom-complex, which is usually already to hand in the inherited disposition, is found mainly in cold, schizoid individuals in whom neurotic overcompensation is also sometimes present. Hence it is present in Frederick the Great, with his inheritance of accumulated, inbred schizoid characters from the house of the Guelphs. Of his four grandparents three were Guelphs, and he thus received an inheritance from queer, eccentric personalities and half-mad schizophrenics which spun itself further into the insane schizophrenic kings of Bavaria, Otto and Louis II.

The inner driving power to uncommon deeds may in this group be derived from sadistic-masochistic mechanisms, which we analysed earlier. The type comes to a fine historical expression in Robespierre, an heroic leader with the coldest schizoid traits and an ethically-sublimated sadism. In some ways he impresses one as an extreme caricature of Frederick the Great. The same essential features stand out : abstract, virtuous idealism ; belief in schemes for a model state, and cruel indifference to individuals and individual fate (" My good fellows, did you expect to live for ever ? ").

From medical sources we know a good deal about Robespierre. His father while still quite young fell into an incurable melancholy. He sought to rid himself of torturing self-reproach by travelling, but all in vain, and four years later he died abroad. In Robespierre himself the most important schizoid symptoms depicted in historical records are the disconnectedness of his bodily movements, the uncontrollable twitching of his shoulders, the stiff machine-like way in which he walked and all the unnatural, false and pedantic qualities in his gestures and modes of expression. From one of the older sketches I select the following excellent characterisation of Robespierre which is well in agreement with the chief features of other historical research monographs :

" The man whom Paris and France made in the first degree responsible for that horror perpetrated in the name of freedom and equality—the man at whose name Royalists and Republicans alike turned pale in their defencelessness, was a gentle, likeable and tender-hearted friend of the house of Duplay, deputy of the committee of public safety : Maximilian Robespierre. Undoubtedly the psychological riddle bound up in the name of Robespierre has never been solved. It is unanimously agreed by members of all parties who were acquainted with the facts that the originator of the reign of terror was not the mean, godless, half-mad tyrant, lacking in all moral sense, that his enemies and conquerors in their hatred and lust for revenge, have depicted. Certainly opponents and supporters alike join in the opinion that Robespierre in his private life was impeccable, that in his outward dealings he was a respectable and honest citizen, that he never made personal profit from his position of power and that he was sincerely convinced of the benefits to be derived from his political system. Mirabeau's remark : ' This man believes everything that he says,' was ever accepted by shrewd contemporaries as the most fitting characterisation of Robespierre, whose reason, becoming colder and more fanatical. had become madness. Napoleon who had close connections with Robespierre's younger brother, spoke of the renowned man of terror in a similar vein to Mirabeau : ' He was a fanatic, a monster, but incorruptible and incapable of endangering anyone's life simply for the sake of personal gain. In these matters he was an honourable man.' On the other hand the best informed of Robespierre's apologists do not deny that the dictator of French public opinion was morose, suspicious, and, in spite of a certain sentimentality, cold and inhuman. They would admit that his pedantic, half-shy, half-disdainful nature was practically lacking in power of attraction, that indeed his concealed irritability awoke aversion, and that the sententious, pompous, prolix and pedantic style of his speeches excluded them from any comparison with the brilliant eloquence of Mirabeau, the fire of Danton or the ideal cadences of the Girondist, Vergniaud. Finally the testimony of all contemporaries is at one in stating that this tremulous coward, cowering before every physical danger, was in other fields a ' giant of will power ' who in strength of character and the boldness of his decisions stood second to none of his rivals.

"But how comes it that a man who lacked all personal attractiveness and any real oratorical talent was able for five years to rise constantly in public estimation and to attain his goals in parliament, in committee, and in the general assembly ? How did he succeed in driving all competitors from the field ? And how is it to be explained that this pedantic, rancorous and affected hypochondriac was regarded by those who lived with him as a paragon of goodness and amiability ; that this gloomy, bookish man, without a spark of gallantry, inspired women of the most varied age and education with idolatrous admiration and tenderness ? Of

L

the outer qualities which are said to please women Robespierre possessed none. Already, when he was only a little
over thirty years old, he made the impression of a dried-up
old bachelor. Of middling height, slim and proportionately
built he strode about as stiffly as a wire doll, his head thrown
back and his arms and legs moving like levers. His manner
was one of assumed gravity and his expression denoted a
studied interest. At a casual glance one saw nothing more
in his face than illness and inward dissatisfaction. But
closer observation betrayed peculiarly-cast, indeed extraordinary, characters. Below the rather low brow, the lines
of which expressed earnestness and deliberation, a pair of
greenish eyes, usually inflamed, looked out from behind the
protection of darkish spectacles. The rather prominent nose,
slightly hooked in the upper part, spoke of unusual self-will
and determination. That he was a sufferer from liver trouble
was plainly indicated by the peculiar brownish-yellow tinge
of his complexion. The firmly-shut lips of his sharply
chiselled mouth writhed convulsively whenever this nervous
being was in any way excited. The whole of his body,
especially his shoulders, would twitch in sympathy and the
studied dignity of his demeanour would be torn to pieces.
When the features of this morose countenance sought to
smile they merely distorted themselves into a grimace, in
which there was no gaiety, but only horror. Robespierre's
voice was powerful but raw and unmodulated and presented
him with many difficulties, which he only succeeded in
mastering towards the end of his career as an orator. By
speech he was often deeply moved and he shed tears during
his own orations, a fact which has quite wrongly been set
down to hypocrisy. Like most cold, detached men who are
busied with themselves and their own ideas, Robespierre

possessed a strongly sentimental vein. The ideas to which he was devoted stamp him as a true child of the sentimental eighteenth century, in spite of some contradictory elements in his character. Robespierre's favourite writer, whom he worshipped and idolised, was Rousseau. 'The Social Contract' was his political Bible and the desire to realise the impracticable schemes of that book, to bring men by force to virtue, simplicity and selfless altruism, was the dream of his life. The 'New Heloise' represented for him the highest ideal of womanhood and the 'Emile' the highest law for the conduct of his private life. Finally, the pathos with which Rousseau set forth his teachings on civil virtue and the truths of nature affected Robespierre as the essence of all poetry.

" Two members of the Duplay family, the father and the youngest daughter, outlived their renowned companion and preserved for his memory an inspired adoration and gratitude to the end of their lives. According to their accounts, this fear-inspiring man of power was in private life the most unassuming, good-natured and tractable of mortals, the favourite alike of children, grown-ups and servants. This is all the more remarkable since Robespierre was otherwise an extraordinarily reserved and abnormally sensitive individual, who turned with fundamental aversion from the fashionable, sansculotte familiarity which had appeared with the revolution."

Robespierre, who had foreseen his downfall for months before it occurred, had nevertheless scorned to attach himself to any definite political party, though that alone could have saved him. In the press of hostile action which gathered around him, escape depended above all on swift tactics and rapid intuition of personal motives and relationships ; but in these things he was a complete failure. He refused to make the final decision to which his friends urged him. Set free, half against his will, he wasted the precious hours with words and hoped to acquit himself by a theatrical speech of explanation.

Having executed so many enemies of his ideal state, with his hand on ' The Social Contract ', and with the pedantic incorruptibility of a schoolmaster, he now found, when the same fate threatened him, that his principles did not permit him to call upon the passions of the mob for rescue. In whose name, he asked himself, had anyone the right to stir the people to revolt against the accepted National Assembly ? And as he knew no answer, he refused to sign what was put before him, thereby giving himself up to execution.

When pedantic adherence to principle ˙ overstrides a certain level it becomes greatness of spirit ; and detachment from the world, occurring at decisive moments, is transformed into the noblest realities of world history. In the seething witch-cauldron of revolutionary Paris, Mirabeau, the most outstanding ' man of the world ' and the cleverest student of human nature in all France, could only assert himself with difficulty. But Robespierre had dominated and con-trolled it for years in its maddest and most catastrophic changes ; Robespierre, a man of books and theories, who thought that with a couple of dozen guillotines he could transform rococo France into an abstract, ideal state ; Robespierre, who all his life long had no notion what a human being is. A biographer has called him ' Principle in the flesh ' and forgotten thereby only that it is impossible to speak of flesh and blood where Robespierre is concerned. The sadism in the foundations of his soul had transformed itself into an abstract ideology of virtue and continued to express itself according to that mould. Apart from that, one cannot discover any living or human thing in him. All the hate of his enemies never succeeded in unearthing the slightest tale of amorous liaisons or immorality in a world which was full of such tales and lived by them. For women he had only aversion or well-bred politeness, and in all respects his private life was without blemish. Among men he had only political associates and admirers, but never a friend. He was indeed a man of impeccable righteousness who paid no attention to persons because for his emotional life there were no persons, only ideas ; a man for whom beauty and pleasure were empty words, who remained unattracted by all that entices living men, who, given limitless power, bestowed upon himself neither wealth nor honours. Robespierre was no man but a virtuous ghost, a monster walking in sleep and without feeling for the monstrous. There are horrifying situations in history, in which a fully conscious, feeling person would become giddy, and through which indeed a sleep-walker alone can pass. Robespierre dreamt of Rousseau's Arcadian state of humanity and with that dream vision before his eyes, he set himself a path, as straight as the flight of a bullet, through the swarm of passionately excited humanity, never noticing what went down before him in his course. Robespierre's dream of Roman virtue was precisely similar to Hölderlin's vision of Greece. But the dream which Hölderlin dreamt among trees and flowers Robespierre dreamt on the driver's seat of the madly-careering coach of state. ˙ And the tones of the Arcadian shepherds' flutes were in truth a signal for the bloodiest destruction.

What, then, is the leader, the masterful man of power ? Robespierre, the sickly, shy, sentimental pedant, represents one of the bloodiest of them.

TENTH CHAPTER

Inspired Characters and Mankind's Veneration

HÖLDERLIN lives on as a tragic figure in the history of literature. Shortly after his thirtieth year the earnest, tender-hearted, over-sensitive poet became a victim of incurable insanity and under the shadows of schizophrenic psychosis he passed away his life in Hölderlin's Tower on the Neckar at Tübingen until, at seventy-three, he died. There one could see him, a pointed white cap upon his head, wandering, irresolute and phantom-like, to and fro, before the window. That sight awoke in Mörike, as a young student, the phantastic romance of the fire rider : " See yonder at the little window the red cap comes again." Many years before the outbreak of the actual psychosis, the emotional coldness and rigidity gradually creeping over him can be perceived in the tones of his poems, from which the horror of the schizophrenic breathes at us, and in which the world and his own living spirit became gradually transformed into an icy world of phantoms.

> " Where art thou ? Life still lingered
> With me as my evening closed coldly,
> And quiet as the shadows I am here,
> My shuddering heart asleep in my bosom."

This feeling of an icy change, of a growing, deep strangeness in all experience, has been recorded by many schizophrenics at the beginning of their psychosis. They have the feeling as if their thoughts are no longer their own, that a strange hand in some magical way has dipped into their spiritual life, that their ideas come from without, now thrust into consciousness, now arbitrarily withdrawn, and that they have become the tool of encroaching powers. Such a belief was that of Schumann, when he was overtaken by mental disease, that the musical motives produced by his over-stimulated brain came to him from angel voices, indeed from Schubert and Mendelssohn in the beyond. He would stand the whole day at his writing-table with music paper before him and listen with glances of profound felicity to what they sang for him.

The threat to the integrity of the personality felt by the patient in his inward experience of the disease process, the fact that " everything is thrown into ruins as by an ex-traneous force," has been projected by the more intellectual schizophrenics with uniform regularity into the cosmos and viewed as a world catastrophe. There arises a compelling sense of great metaphysical connections, a profound oneness with the universe and with godliness. Everything is bril-liantly lit up, clear as the edge of a precipice, and strangely threatening. Recoiling from a state of horrible fear into one of ecstatic rapture, the patient now believes in his own annihilation, in a twilight of the gods, in weirdly threatening catastrophes and the destruction of all the world, from which he will arise like a phoenix from the ashes, as saviour, as prophet, indeed as God and Christ Himself, to lead forth his fellow-men to renewed life. Like the mystic he perceives a constant interplay of microcosm with macrocosm, sees everywhere unexpected relations, strange, dreadful, en-chanting connections. He has the last and deepest insight into the decrees of God, sees the planets weaving in obscure symbolical designs the fate of mortals, and believes that his personal sins, his erotic impulses, his salvation, are wrapt up in the same cosmic movements and accompanied by magical influence. And for him all old things are past; everything is reborn.

This feeling of sudden and complete inversion of personality, of being overpowered by some alien influence, of a destruction of the boundaries of the self with assimilation to the infinite, can be of the greatest moment if the schizophrenic process does not progress to the ultimate spiritual catastrophe, but only far enough to leave behind a peculiarly transformed, autistic, world-shy, fanatical or enthusiastic personality. Precisely this devastating experience of inspiration and conversion, this overpowering feeling of being gripped in the elemental depths of one's soul by a supernatural power, can be the starting-point, if awakened in a strong personality, of great changes in world history. Principally this experience of inspiration has led to monumental reconstruction in the realm of religion. How far such processes played a part with the great founders of religion it is difficult to say, for their personalities are wrapt in the mists of superstition and tradition.

The same powerfully-emotional, intrusive experience of extreme metaphysical ecstasy is also found among epileptics, generally in the moments preceding an attack. The epileptic Dostoievsky has described it with great truth to nature in his novels : " It is a matter of seconds, altogether not more than five or six, in which one feels suddenly the one, eternal harmony which fills all existence. There is no longer anything earthly here. I do not say that it is heavenly ; I only say that man as an earthly being cannot bear it. One must become physically transformed—or die. It is as if one suddenly felt the whole of nature within himself and said,

' Yes, that is truth.'   Be on your guard, Kiriloff—that is
an attack of epilepsy coming ! "   Think of Mahomet who
on his horse flew through the whole of heaven before the
water had run out of the jug, the jug emptied itself in five
seconds—and Mahomet was an epileptic.

Figures which stand in historical twilight, as that of
Mahomet, cannot be regarded by the psychiatrist as suitable
personalities for analysis.   It is, however, well known that
the apostle Paul suffered from a complaint commonly
believed to have been epilepsy.   According to his own
accounts he had one chronic burden, an arrow in his flesh,
and we know too of his ecstasy before Damascus which led
to his conversion, in which he was gathered to the seventh
heaven and cast down.   It is no accident that an inclination
to religion is particularly encountered among schizophrenics
and epileptics.   The relation is so regular and definite that
even a modern philosopher has supposed an especially close
interconnection of metaphysics with schizophrenic conditions
of mind.   These sufferers from mental disturbance have
religious experiences in their acute conditions which are
deeper, more catastrophic and more compelling than those
of hysterics.   But the latter are the chief actors in miraculous
healings, stigmatisation and religious epidemics.   And, among
the first class, the schizophrenic experiences of inspiration
have naturally played a more important rôle in history than
the more uniform, less spiritually differentiated, states of
epileptics.

Disease, mystic ecstasy and distressing poverty hover
in the dark shadowy records of the origins of religion, its
founders and its saints.   The poor in spirit, the mentally
diseased, found the kingdom of heaven.   The healthy and
strong made out of it a system and a power.   But all alike

speak with conviction, as if with absolute knowledge, of the transcendental. Which is the true voice from the beyond ? Is it the frenzied tones of ecstatic schizophrenics, of frothing epileptics, of howling dervishes, or the hollow chants of monks singing their psalms in loneliness ? Or is it the precise and pointed discourse of philosophers and the solemn bene-dictions of wise high priests ? Everyone of them calls to himself with his own echo in vast reverberating space. They believe that the metaphysical essence talks to them or wraps them round in a great silence.

The poet Hölderlin, with his sensitive, tender, emotional disposition, so needful of protection, had a deeply religious nature. Even late in the years of his insanity he one day asked his guardian, Zimmer the cabinet-maker, to construct for him a Greek temple out of wood, and then he wrote on a piece of board :

" Most varied are the lines of life.
Oh, how the paths wind and the mountains end.
But whatsoever we are here, God will later complete,
With his rewards, eternal harmony and peace."

Already in his years of sanity Hölderlin's spirits were almost constantly wounded by this and that. Inwardly he could never bridge the deep chasm which separated the artistic dreams of his proud, sensitive soul from the coarse, brutal realities of the world of men. But his fine feeling for spiritual independence would never permit him to find satisfaction for his inner need of ' harmony and peace ' in the teachings of the church.

Thus it came about that his religious feelings found their characteristic expression in a deep, impassioned pantheism, which, from his youth, continued to be the fundamental note of his personality and his poetry. The inner foundations of his mystical love of nature he himself revealed in an ode : ' Caprices ' :

"Beneath the shadows of the forest, where the mighty sun
Of noon, glimmers softly through the foliage,
I sit quietly, alone,
When, angry with many insults,

I have wandered forth into the wild—thy poets,
Nature, are angry all too easily. They mourn and weep so readily
These blessed ones ; like children
Whom the mother presses too tenderly.

They are ill-tempered and full of masterful self-will ;
If they follow the path quietly for a time, yet
Soon they go astray ; they fling themselves
Away from the path, struggling with thee.

Yet thou scarcely touchest them, loving one ; with kindness
They are happy and good ; they cheerfully obey,
Thou guidest them, oh, Mistress Mother,
With gentle reins, wherein thou willst."

In this ode Hölderlin, deeply wounded by mankind, flees beneath the tree-tops, opening his inmost heart to the gentle guidance and protection of nature to which, as to a mother, he had an entirely personal, childlike, pious relationship. A god saved him from ' the noise and torment of men.' " I understood the ethereal stillness ; but human words I never understood. I was brought up by the sweet voices of the rustling groves and learnt to love among the flowers. In the arms of the gods I came to manhood." Schizoid persons are usually very serious and Hölderlin, too, was an entirely humourless nature. Not only was he autistically over-sensitive towards the impressions of real human life but he also lacked the capacity to reconcile these impressions by an inner synthesis. In social intercourse he was quite incapable of appreciating the slightest joke. He was suspicious of the most casual remarks made in his presence and a slight smile was able to disturb him and make him feel " degraded in his inmost sanctuary." Hence his strained, idealistic conception of human intercourse caused him to sway constantly between the ecstasies of passionate cults of friendship and the most despondent disillusionment and bitterness. His feeling of strangeness and fear in face of reality he described in the following words : " I almost think that I am precise and pedantic out of love itself. I am not shy out of fear of being disturbed by reality in self-absorption, but I am afraid that reality will intrude into my inmost interests with which I try to attach myself to outside things. I am fearful of having the warm life within me frozen by the ice-cold stream of daily events."

In that passage Hölderlin has expressed what is felt fundamentally by all finely-endowed schizoids in face of the real instinctive life of men. A man of this sort, who can so easily be mortally wounded by a passing joke, is never able to feel at home with mankind as a whole, however much he may be given to tender, exaggerated individual friendships. Just as the schizoid who is lacking in feeling withdraws into himself and presents the aspect of a morose, misanthropic eccentric, so the artistic, feeling schizoid, with his inmost need of consideration and love, flees anywhere where his delicate phantasies will receive no opposition or hurt through the will of other men. Thus he escapes into some idealised era of the past, into the realm of artistic life or books, but especially into the beauty of nature where it is untouched by man. Out of this need to find some substitute for human life as the object of affection and emotional expression, arise with smaller minds all those innumerable hobbies and whimsical partialities so characteristic of old bachelors and eccentrics and so lacking in any human element. The painter Spitzweg, himself inclined to this disposition, has painted a delicious collection of such types : the cactus lover, the cultivator of carnations, the bee farmer, the star gazer, the collector of rare objects and the bookworm.

But Hölderlin, the genius, as an asylum from the inclemency of the coarse and hostile realities of humanity, built for himself from his fondest day-dreams the temple of his final philosophy, in which the gods of Greece dwelt side by side with Mother Nature and Father Ether. It was an elegant temple, of classical purity of style, but its lines were softened by the tender, mystic twilight of romanticism. Himself, and the few people he loved, he felt to be Hellenes who had strayed into a raw, later age. His brothers, whom he sought in vain among his fellow-men, he found eventually in the Athens of Pericles among the ideal figures of his imagination. And the clear blue sky of Hellas became for him a kind of godhead, Father Ether, who, in tranquillity and goodness, blessed all men and was the inner essence of infinite, all-comprehending, all-loving Nature. All the figures that lived in Hölderlin's phantasies and moved through his poems were of a quiet, saintly beauty. Nowhere is loud reality ; everywhere the personified feelings of the poet himself, and the soft, veiled inner light of his autistic, delicately emotional personality. Whatsoever he was to love and worship must have fine lines, and whatsoever he found beautiful, to that he prayed. Religion and poetry for him are thus melted into one ; his poetic art and his philosophy of life become a single, delicate and totally unreal system. His pious adoration of Nature satisfies the most personal, intimate feelings of love. Therein his inner being is drawn to every tree, flower and cloud, because they, like schizophrenic persons are quiet, dreamy and lonely and, unlike the world of men, do not know how to hurt and wound.

Hölderlin's novel, "Hyperion," is also a picture like a dream island, timeless and without action. Figures that are never human beings but only transparent, tender shapes of desire, float before one without any will of their own in the cadence of a language that is really music. They drift to and fro, and weave out of the discords of the world, with the two magic words, Nature and Hellas, a harmony for which the unhappy poet had longed all his life in vain.

For schizoids, contact with the realities of human life is dissonance, and harmony is found only in the dreamy beauty of inanimate nature. Hence the essential pantheism which calls to us from "Hyperion" was for him a release from reality, and a pouring out of his love for all that which he was still able to love:

"You springs of earth! You flowers! Forests, eagles and friendly light! How old and new is our love! We are free and do not need to compare ourselves anxiously from without! How then shall life not change? We love the boundless ether and become one in the inmost essence. Oh, Spirit; beauty of the world! Thou art: what then is death and all the sorrows of humanity? Ah, many inanimate words, together, have made the miraculous. In the end everything is done from joy and finishes with peace. The discords of the world are but the quarrels of lovers. Reconciliation comes in the midst of battle and all separated things find each other again."

ELEVENTH CHAPTER

The Prophet

" I AM commencing a work which has no precedent and will find no imitators. I will draw for my fellow-men a human being, true to nature in all parts, and that being— am I. I alone. I am not made like any other living person. I may not be better, but I am at least different. The trump of doom may ring out when it will ; I shall tread before the Highest Judge, with this book in my hand, and say in a loud voice : ' Here is what I have created, what I have thought, what I have been. Gather my brothers around me, let them listen to my confessions, sigh over my infamies and blush for my weaknesses. Let every one of them open his heart with the same truthfulness at the foot of Thy throne, and if then there be one among them who still dares, let him step forward undisturbed and say, " I was a better being than this man." ' "

The man who opened the story of his life with these words suffered from delusions of persecution. It was the French philosopher Rousseau, one of the intellectual creators of the great French Revolution. Another time he wrote : " There may be people who dislike my books and I do not blame them for it ; but whoever reads my books and dislikes me—is a knave."

Thus speaks the man who, as a boy at school, lied, stole and played truant ; who deserted almost all his patrons, led the life of a homeless adventurer, lived with a plebeian landlady without marrying her and sent his five children to a foundling hospital. Was he perhaps right in all this ?

When Schiller saw the young Hölderlin for the first time he couched his opinion in the following expression : " What an intense subjectivity he has." The same intense subjectivity speaks out of every one of the introductory sentences of Rousseau's " Confessions." Both men, Hölderlin and Rousseau, loved above all things a limitless independence of inward and outward conditions, and loved it at the price of hunger and homelessness. Rousseau, the copier of music, trembled for his independence when offered a good living, just as much as did the tutor Hölderlin.

There is a kind of self-regard which has its roots in an all too great spiritual delicacy : people who are proud in that way we call highly-strung, sensitive personalities. At the bottom of their natures lies a weakness of vitality, a vulnerability and an over-sensitivity in relation to everyday happenings. When the struggle goes against them they have no strength on which to call, but they can still summon up the pride which ennobles their weaknesses. Rousseau had many sides to his character which were incompatible ; among other things, he was a conscientious man. For what he did as a Bohemian, he could not, as a moralist, be responsible. If he was too refined and noble for a careless, witty vagabond, he was equally too naïve for a moralist. The violent tension in sensitive souls between their pride and their weakness, is the spring of their spiritual greatness and the rock of their intellectual vitality. The most powerful spiritual forces arise like the power of steam from fire and water, from the struggle of hostile elements, from irreconcilable contrasts, that stand at odds within the breast of one and the same person. For that reason the sensitive man, in spite of his weakness, can outgrow socially, the healthy being who has indeed strength but possesses no contrasts.

The greatest reformers have been shy, retiring men. The sensitive person is extremely easily wounded by those tiny discords of life which the healthy person does not even notice. And because of his gentle and constrained nature, he is unable to disembarrass himself forthwith by forceful dealings with the torturing influences. So he becomes the man of inner conflicts, who undergoes constant and severe struggles of conscience for long periods without any outsider being aware of them. And if, at last, fearfully and with many torturing doubts, he has given voice to that which he believes, then probably he shrinks back horrified before the threatening reverberations which his timid utterance has awakened in the masses of the people. Thus it was with that shy, awkward vagrant, Rousseau, who did not know what to do with himself in company, and with the boorish monk, Luther, of the dark, burning glance, who, with coarse outbursts of laughter and smutty abuse, covered up his inner anguish and uncertainty. Their whispered confessions of personal belief become, in the twinkling of an eye, the clamorous war-cries of a century, and the unseen man of learning, or artist, is thrust forward by the passions of his supporters, to an active position of leadership, against which his shy sensitiveness stands inwardly in acute opposition.

The echo of a profound personal experience may set off the explosive emotions of a corrupt age. Rousseau was among the first gusts of the storm, the heralds of the French Revolution, which his intellect had helped to set in motion. But the reins which slipped from his hands were taken up by others. As his writings became famous, he reacted just as one would expect a shy man to react, who is suddenly

M

thrust from his hiding-place into the midst of many people. He felt all eyes directed upon him, and had the strange feeling that everything depended upon him. Then, he could no more preserve himself from the scornful hissing of his enemies, which sounded sharper to his ears than any bursts of applause. It came to him from all sides, like the schemes of a common plot, the close, inescapable meshes of a net of intrigue which was being fastened about his head. Thus arose Rousseau's delusion of persecution, the deeper roots of which we have still to study, which drove him restlessly from Paris to Switzerland, from Switzerland to England, and back again from England to France. It gave him no pause in any haven or with any protecting patron, because, sooner or later, in the most remote hiding-place or lonely castle, he scented a hostile play of forces about him ; the servants seemed to look at him in a strange way, they vexed him and jeered at him, or people spoke of him as a poisoner and wished to take his life : in short, there was a plotting hand constantly working against him, and hunting him from one place of refuge to another. This is the typical systematised delusion of the sensitive person who stands in conflict with himself, and consequently, with his environment.

Why did not the mailed fist of Ulrich von Hutten break open the door to the new age ? Why did the sarcastic Voltaire, master of satire, fail to bring a flush to the face of France in the old régime ? Certainly these were men of the greatest historical effectiveness. They were men who had the ambition to be the leaders of their age at all costs. Hutten had called tirelessly to the people in the German language. His slogan rang out, stirring and defiant : ' I have dared it.' But the masses did not rise up to support him. Yet the involved monkish Latin, that a world-shy cleric had composed in fear and trembling, for his learned colleagues, in the castle church of Wittenberg, ran in a few days to the furthest corners of Europe.

And when the shy dreamer, and planless dilettante, Rousseau, at last in his thirty-seventh year, busied himself to write an academic prize essay on the question, " Has the progress of science and art contributed to the decline or the purification of morals ? " France held its breath in astonishment.

In the gardens and dales of his Swiss home, the youthful Rousseau, happy and full of dreams in spite of a hundred minor fits of temper and foolish actions, lived under the protection of his motherly mistress, knowing no duties as a citizen, neglected, defying the police and withal innocent and planless. He had the tender soul of a child, which men accepted as good even when he deceived them, and which, with overflowing affection, tried to embrace the whole world.

From his going to Paris, arose his greatness and his madness. He was but a Bohemian jack-of-all-trades, and he trotted into Paris like a lamb into a cage of snakes. He stood with the sincere wondering eyes of a child, among the most frivolous cavaliers, spiteful men of letters and experienced scoundrels of his century. When his friend of that time, the philosopher Diderot, sat in prison at Vincennes, Rousseau walked faithfully every day, for two hours, through the burning summer heat, to see him. Waiting outside to see him on his first visit, he was nearly overcome with joy and impatience. " What an inexpressible moment," wrote Rousseau in his " Confessions " : " As I entered, I noticed only him. A spring and a cry was all ; I pressed my face to his, embraced him tightly. I spoke to him only through my sighs and tears and nearly choked with tenderness and

M*

joy." Diderot turned calmly to the priest standing by, and said, " You see, sir, how my friends love me." This little scene is entirely symbolical of the way in which Rousseau flung himself on the breasts of the Parisian men of culture, and of the way they reacted to it. Rousseau's outburst of friendship, finds Diderot, the man of the world, entirely cool and prepared ; in joking about it to those around, he is using him cleverly for his own ends. The jealousy of Voltaire, in matters touching his literary fame was much too great to allow him any beneficial relations with Rousseau. But on the whole, one cannot say that Parisian society encountered Rousseau in any unfriendly spirit. On the contrary he was taken into the best circles ; the drawing-rooms of clever, intellectual women gathered around him ; his gauche eccentricity was not upsetting, indeed his naïveté was felt to be charming and it brought the man of feeling into fashion straight away. Learned men, artists, women and cavalierly gentlemen, soon treated him as one of themselves, and began, as was their habit, to play with him a little and intrigue. For life had indeed become for Rococo-France, a game. One lived on malicious mischief, the scandal of artistic cliques ; one was amused best of all, by pretty frivolities, and little infidelities, and really no serious harm was done to anybody.

Here Rousseau showed himself to be abnormal. He took life, so to speak, literally. When his friend Grimm, gently dispossessed him of the favour of his women patrons, he experienced it as a really mean action, and when the philosopher, Hume, procured for him a kingly pension with one hand, whilst indicating his enjoyment of the satire of envious persons with the other, that was, for Rousseau, a downright breach of faith. That is how Rousseau became the rediscoverer of simple, natural morals. For in good society, of the eighteenth century, it was tasteless to experience things in that way. And only a man with the abnormally-sensitive character structure of Rousseau could think of awakening that attitude again, for here was a man in whom that attitude still lived, as part of his inmost feelings, despite the powerful suggestion to the contrary emanating from the whole outlook of society.

Out of this 'intense subjectivity' of Rousseau, out of this passionate integrity, sprang his struggle with the old order. His cry of ' back to nature ' was given the convincing ring of a personal experience, by the fact that he had encountered in the flesh, the pernicious falseness of a hot-house civilisation in his dealings with his friends. But, from this same root of his Parisian experiences, grew his delusion of persecution. He could not conceive how anyone could help another, and insult him in the same breath. Therefore, his all-too-deep and sensitive nature, supported by the lively combinatory power of his highly-developed brain, suspected a scheming plot in every incidental little quarrel of a literary clique. He, himself, could only feel deeply and inwardly, and he was quite unable to comprehend moods which were only skin deep. Before the mentality of these hardened men of the world, he stood helpless, as before a locked door. The rapidly changing colours of their sentiments, and their constant changes of front, confused his feelings. Where he expected affectionate friendship, he was met with the prick of a needle, and where unbending hostility glowered at him, he was suddenly surprised to find a thoroughly amiable countenance. Whether he went to France or to England it was always the same story. Until, at last, he went mad from their friendliness and their needle-

pricks, and concluded that a system of the most refined
cruelty and spite had been engineered against his person.
He saw a web of subterranean hostile relations spun through
all lands, where, in truth, there were only the passing moods
of envious literary men playing their habitual game. Therefore, the leading spirits of literary life, Grimm and Diderot,
Voltaire and Hume stood in the centre of his insane ideas.
Into their hands he believed all the threads were gathered,
that tightened about his head. He hated the culture of
his time, and he hated the leaders of that culture. The
first led to his works of genius ; the second to his insanity.
His delusion of persecution, and his greatness as a prophet,
are two aspects of the same entity.

At the same time, it must not be forgotten, that real
and sincere injustices were not lacking in Rousseau's life.
People used him to their own ends, and planned mischief
with his manuscripts. When the '' Emile '' was appearing,
Rousseau, threatened with imprisonment, had to flee from
Paris, and he had hardly found sanctuary on Peter's island,
when the Government of Berne turned him out, and the
mob, incited to violence, harassed the gentle, sensitive man
with stone throwing. Thus, objective persecution was not
absent from Rousseau's life. But persecution alone does not
make a delusion of persecution. Neither could the little
malicious actions of literary men, and their frivolous intrigues
have done so ; they might have made him perplexed, bitter,
suspicious and lonely, but they could not have driven him
to that passionate inner conviction, which gave such compelling power to his work of philosophical reform, and
hardened his feeling of persecution into the systematic fixed-
ness of insanity.

The third, deepest and most obscure root of his genius,

and his mental disease lay where it always lies with sensitive men : in the feeling of self-reproach. Rousseau did not believe that he could live through the culture which he despised without being affected by it. He was far removed from that simple, strict virtue of ancient Rome, which floated before him as the true ideal. With his altogether impressionable, lively and hot-blooded, artistic nature, he was much more a child of the kaleidoscopic realities of his own day. Therein lies an essential part of his greatness. He was not like most moralists, like, *e.g.* Robespierre, himself an exponent of a system of dry, abstract virtue, a person who did not sin because he lacked the capacity of sinning : rather, he was one who fought against what he had himself experienced. This dual nature, makes him an especially lovable being, for it was always the basis of his judgment of others, and enabled him to meet the meanest evil with some remnant of his sunny smile. His presence transformed the most doubtful figures, without causing any permanent alteration of his own nature. He could be dragged down for years in the toils of the maddest whirlpool and come to the surface again, with the same unadulterated, childlike spirit. And he understood, too, like the moralists, how to construct his system of philosophy in abstraction, over the head of reality. But, what is more remarkable, he could do both that, and the complete opposite : he enjoyed life while he despised it ; he understood reality and loved it tenderly, while he demonstrated its impossibility. That is the main contrast in his nature, which makes it contradictory and therefore full of genius, and which makes possible the judgment of Schopenhauer, when he remarked of Rousseau, that nature had given him the gift to be able to moralise without becoming a bore.

Rousseau's feeling of guilt and self-reproach, was rooted in his experiences. His experiences were rooted in the depths of his disposition, in the contradictions of instinct within his constitution. There, can be found all the infantilism, the boundless naïveté, the defiant and timid spirit of a child. He remained constantly attached to a mother image ; his erotic tendencies drew him always to elderly, protective women, to whose lap he fled, to Madame de Warens, to Madame d'Epinay. The mother, is for him, mistress, and his mistress, he calls Mama. Or again, he loves the simple woman with no intellect, of whom he used to be nervous and fearful and before whom he used to blush— the woman who later became his wife.

His friendships with men, retained the idealistic, warmly affectionate features of adolescence. These friendships overheated his social intercourse only to leave it colder afterwards. They were one of the chief causes of his disappointments and uncertainties, his suspicions, and finally his madness. He demanded intensely, that men love him, and, at the best, respect him ; and when they only respected him, he became convinced they hated him. Later, he had the strange habit of wearing long Oriental clothes, from which one may well conclude some tendency to dress up in feminine garments. But, the masochistic and exhibitionistic traits, have been clearly described by himself, and play a significant rôle in his youthful experiences, in which, he had pleasure in being beaten, and being stripped. These subsidiary instinctive lines of his nature, can be continuously seen, in sublimated, intellectualised forms, at later periods of his life, mainly in his attraction to martyr rôles, which he would readily slide into, or, failing that, provoke. Especially are they expressed in the reckless self-revelation of his personal life, so marked in his " Confessions " : it is precisely this trait, which, in the end, we have to thank for the unusually profound knowledge of his spiritual structure which we possess.

With such conflicting instincts within, it is impossible to keep a straight path. Whichever he followed, the opposing instincts would make him appear false, dishonourable, or mean. He would have to tread any path as a guilty, reproached person, running against the laws of nature, and the commands of his own disposition. His attitude to life, must remain uncertain, burdened with embarrassing failures, against which an intense desire for esteem and a position of respect would have to raise its head all the more obstinately.

That out of this contradiction in his personality, a remainder was left over, is only to be expected. This remainder, is the feeling of guilt of the sensitive idealist, as he gazes back, in pained astonishment, at the confused zigzag which reality has made out of his strivings. The feeling of guilt, turned the second half of his life into a period of genius, which transformed the suffering of retrospection into the passionate pathos of a programme of the future. The same feeling of guilt, however, formed the beginning of his persecution mania, in which, he ascribed to the supposed intrigues of his enemies, all the things which tormented him within himself. That he had sent his children to a foundling hospital, that he had been made to appear insincere in his love to his protectress, Madame d'Epinay, that he had not been able to maintain, in the midst of the entangled scheming of the cunning and ambitious seekers of power, that constancy and faith in friendship which he held to be the highest good ; all these things, which, in reality, plagued only his own conscience, seemed to him, in his insanity, the material which his enemies were eagerly exploiting. That imperishable work, the account of his life, was written under the dominance of his madness, and presents nothing less than the reasoned defence of a paranoiac against his supposed enemies. And, because, at the root of his delusion, there lay a feeling of guilt, that story of his life bore the title " Confessions ".

In so far as Rousseau was a being of highly sensitive feelings—and that was, perhaps, the greater half of his personality—he is similar, even in the finest details, to the schizophrenic Hölderlin. His delicate, sensitive emotionality, repelled by harsh reality, fled back to the calm greatness of the men of antiquity and unspoilt nature, and for Rousseau, as for Hölderlin, the worship of these entities became religion.

But for the melancholy Hölderlin, that reverence was founded in pessimism, flight and a weary looking-back on something that could never return ; whereas for Rousseau, these things were living ideals, worthy of great effort, in a better, future age. For Hölderlin, they spelt resignation ; for Rousseau, a programme. Rousseau, full of easy-flowing, effervescent, intellectual life, looked at the world with optimism. He had something of the nature of a true musician, indeed, he had had great success in Paris as a composer of opera. It sounds almost incredible that this sunny, sanguine nature, could dwell in the same breast with the sensitive, heavy earnestness of the rest of his soul. One of nature's strange caprices of inheritance, had brought into existence, this singularly-contrasting, bizarre personality. Side by side with his tender vulnerability, Rousseau had inherited a good measure of the light-hearted, easy-going, artistic temperament of his father, a widely travelled man, who lived to enjoy life. It was this mercurial temperament which enabled him to recover with astounding elasticity, from the heaviest blows of fate. His irrestrainable imagination went to the utmost limits in all things, as he remarked in a letter to Malesherbes. But, scarcely had some adverse situation brought him to the edge of madness, when, just as everyone was thinking him deadly unhappy, and prostrated with depression, there would turn up from some obscure hiding-place, a bunch of the most charming letters, letters which he had evidently written in the most amiable mood, and which breathed the peace of the country muses and the quiet happiness of his soul. Thus, shortly after the agitation of his escape from Paris, he began, in the diligence which bore him on his flight, to take up once more the translation of Gessner's idylls. The boyhood of the little vagabond Rousseau, was full of careless joys, of unfettered ramblings and an inconsequent snatching at all the brightly-coloured soap bubbles of the moment. " Remote prospects," said Rousseau of himself, " have rarely had any strong influence on my actions. The future is uncertain : all plans which stretch far into the future, I have always regarded as the bait of fools. The smallest delight that can be attained straight away, appeals to me more than all the joys of paradise." The honourable position in a highly respectable family of Savoy to which, as a youthful adventurer, he had successfully attained and which opened to him the most brilliant prospects, he threw away, to go merrily wandering without money or shelter over the Alps, with a street urchin of Geneva, whose face appealed to him. A parlour trick with which he amused the servants, was his only means of livelihood, and when it went wrong and could be used no more, his happiness was all the greater. With his head full of the most excellent castles in the air, he strolled unconcernedly through the magnificent mountain scenery, whilst his clothes and shoes fell to pieces. He was, in turn, musician, lay-brother in a monastery, apprentice, page, jack-of-all-trades, and street boy, according to what entered his head, to-day hungry and roofless, to-morrow, the darling of fine women, gaily chattering at the tables of rich merchants and barons. Finally he landed with Madame de Warens, the good fairy and saint, protectress of beggars, adventurers and talented vagabonds. She was his mother, his mistress, his wife, whom he dearly loved, a soul as good-natured and unpractical, as capricious and inconstant, as frivolous and lovable as himself. Together they squandered their means, and after many adventures retired into the country to Les Charmettes, a wild, overgrown abode in the secluded corner of a valley, with a splashing brook, chestnut woods and terraced garden. Therewith, began the brief, happiest period of his life in a simple rural paradise. When he was writing things down, as an old man, and thought of that time, all the magic of youth would come back to him. " Towards the end of summer, when we slept there for the first time, I felt beside myself with joy. ' O Mama,' I cried, as with tears I gathered her in my arms, ' here is happiness ; here is innocence. If we both do not find it here, we need never trouble to look anywhere else for it.' "

The dreams of poets and philosophical systems are wish-fulfilments. The youthful Rousseau, with a heart full of bold plans and beautifully simple theories, was drawn to Paris, and Paris made him old and unhappy. Rousseau, the old man, after a life of travel, fame and splendour, looked back longingly out of his embitterment, at the youthful Rousseau, who with nothing—was entirely happy. But to return : out of this wish, sprang Rousseau's philosophical system, which was to lead men back again, out of the glaring evils of their civilisation, to the simple paradise of childhood, where there were only innocent shepherds and tillers of the soil, and no law other than that of benevolent Mother Nature.

This brotherly paradise of men which Rousseau painted, and which is still the guiding star of many souls, took its charm from the lost days of youth, from the blue mountains of Savoy and the garden of Charmettes.

PART III
PORTRAIT COLLECTION

PRELIMINARY REMARKS ON THE
ILLUSTRATIONS

THE following collection of portraits provides mainly the material under discussion in the third chapter. It shows, in a number of statistical series, the regular correspondences between the type of intellectual performance and the general physical form; that is, it demonstrates the fundamental biological laws of personality. The standpoint from which these portraits have been gathered, and according to which they must be judged, has been fully developed in my book on 'Physique and Character'. The historical portrait material has been carefully examined, compared and critically selected. In order not to swell the series beyond all bounds I have appended only a few well-accented selections to this book. In the realm of research into genius, it is nowhere possible to produce a statistical series, free of all gaps, because, at the border-lines between the characteristic mental groups, one's judgment becomes uncertain. But it suffices here, as in biology generally, if we can demonstrate characteristic differences in the frequency of distribution, *i.e.* very plentiful or very meagre relationships between various statistical groups. For that purpose, our material is entirely adequate, even if we take into consideration all the sources of error in the handing-down of portraits through history, and all the uncertainties connected with single controversial cases. The correspondence between physique and direction of talent is similar in men of genius to that which we have shown, by extensive series of experiments, to exist among normal men. As far as age is concerned, most of our portraits are pictures at middle age or mature years. Hence, in the main, they offer safely comparable groups of approximately similar age. A few isolated youthful pictures are interspersed, mostly among the lyric poets and dramatists, but even if they were omitted, the statistical results would not be affected.

When we examine the individual groups according to the nature of their intellectual activities, we notice that the philosophers show an astonishingly marked predominance of members of the leptosomatic types of physique, mostly in the normal, pure type, with narrow, sharply-cut features, but also in variations towards infantilism (Kant) and dysplasia (Nietzsche). Athletic features are rarely seen, but perhaps they are most strongly represented in Hegel, Fichte and Hamann. Pyknic types among the great names of philosophy are extremely rare after the sixteenth century. A fully developed pyknic physique, as far as I can see, is nowhere to be detected, and definite pyknic elements are only to be seen in Schelling.

On the other hand pyknics, and types with a strong pyknic alloy, are easily found, in large numbers and leading positions, among the men who have been great naturalists. These are men, who showed in the highest degree a talent for true empiricism, *i.e.* the greatest capacity for concrete observation through the senses : seeing, hearing, and tasting, all of which are so necessary to exact truth-to-nature in description. Proceeding thence, to the mathematico-physical wing of science, *i.e.* towards abstract science, one observes the pyknic element to decline and the leptosomes to increase. In the whole realm of natural science and medicine, one finds all kinds of complicated mixtures of talent, as indeed, the subject demands. In fact there are, between the two wings of science, numerous mixtures of bodily build, as one would expect. Pyknic forms are especially frequent (but in no way exclusive) among the classical figures of biological science (Botany, Zoology, Bacteriology, etc.), and also, in a large group of medical men famous for clinical work. It is no accident, that, in addition, the two patriarchs of popular materialism in the nineteenth century (Vogt and Moleschott) were pyknics. The two brothers Humboldt, I have purposely put close together, because they constitute an especially beautiful example of a divergence of mental type paralleled by a precisely corresponding diverge of anatomical structure. Similar, clear correspondences between direction of talent and bodily form, are found among men of letters. Pyknic portraits are outstandingly frequent among the masters of broad, colourful, realistic prose style, and warm, realistic humour. This literary section is, indeed, almost purely pyknic in physique. Equally marked, is the frequent appearance of leptosomes among dramatists, writers of tragedy, romanticists and artists of pure style. These, like the philosophers again, show a few variants towards dysplasia (Grabbe, Fr. Schlegel) and infantilism (Kleist) but athletic types are once more very rare.

Leptosomes and pyknics form numerically the greatest part, and the most clearly defined types, in the realm of intellectual performances which rank as genius, whilst athletics and the severely dysplastic, abnormally-developed physiques are more weakly represented.

The selection of portraits for illustration in this book, was not made according to eminence of talent, nor simply according to the accepted grouping of historical literature, but according to their appertenance to certain typical forms of intellectual productivity, which we know to be representative of definite clinical types of physical constitution.

We hope, that in addition to illustrating these fundamental biological results, our collection of pictures will be of interest to those studying individual personalities and their intellectual expressions.

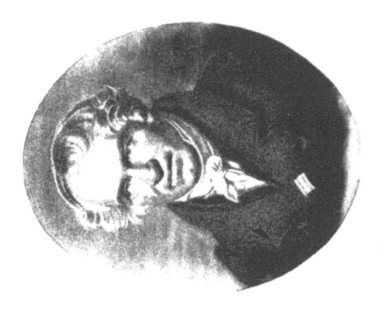

ALEXANDER VON HUMBOLDT

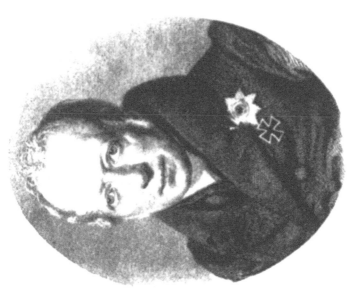

WILHELM VON HUMBOLDT

I. PHILOSOPHERS

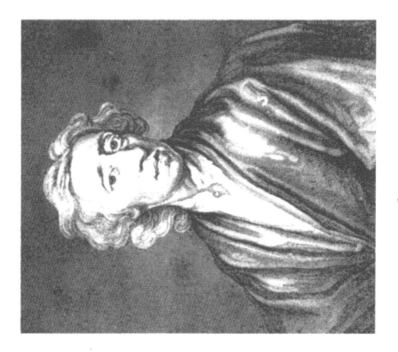

LOCKE

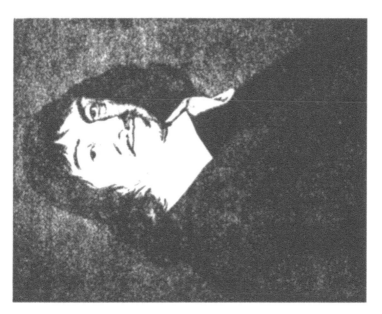

DESCARTES

201

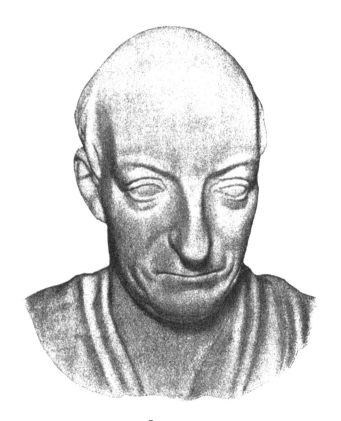

Leibniz

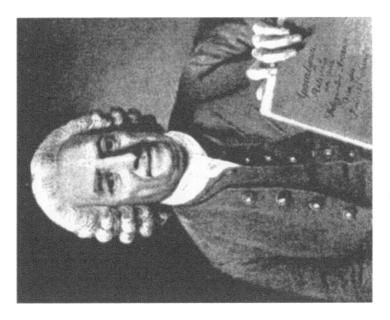

SWEDENBORG

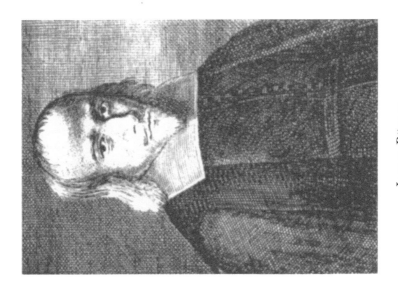

JAKOB BÖHME

203

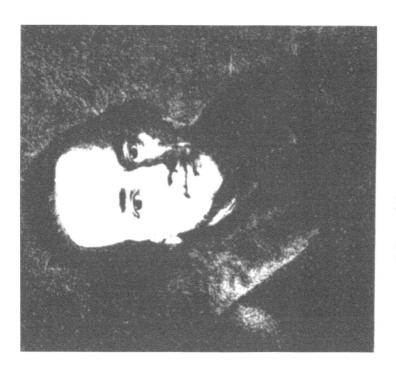

MOSES MENDELSSOHN

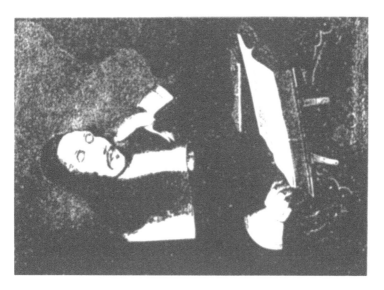

SPINOZA

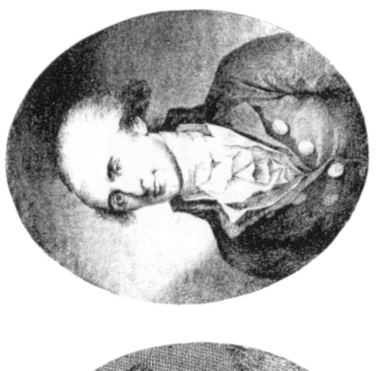

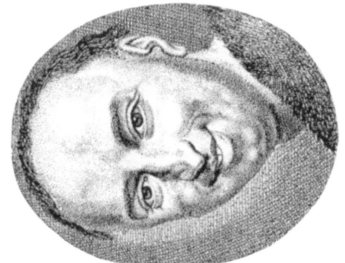

JAKOBI

LA METTRIE

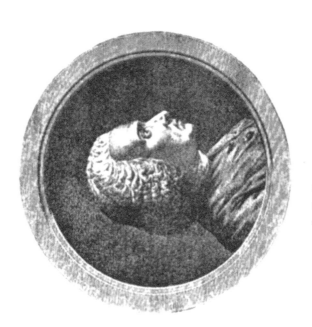

Voltaire

J. J. Rousseau

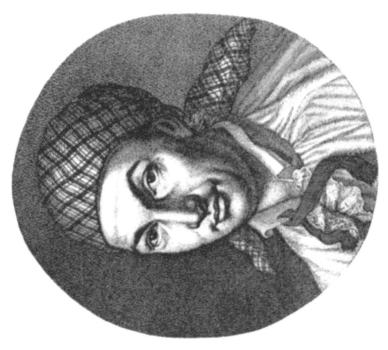

HAMANN

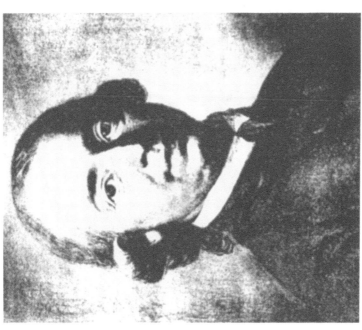

HERDER

207

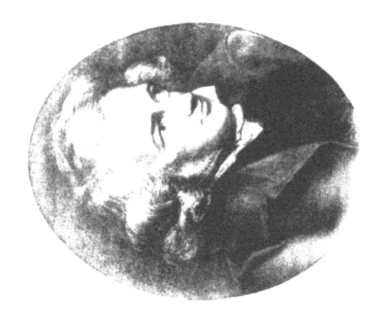

SCHLEIERMACHER

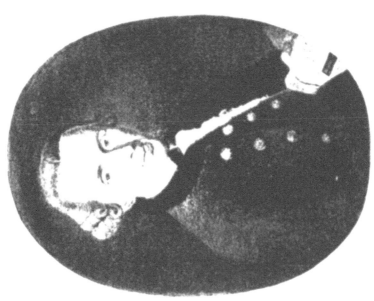

KANT

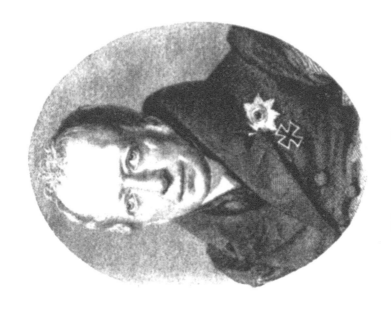

WILHELM VON HUMBOLDT

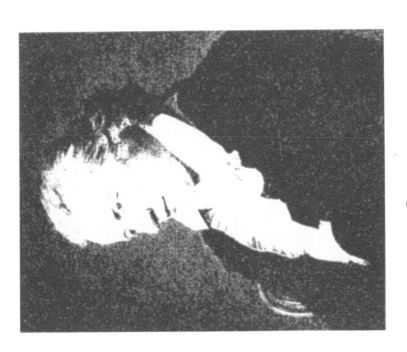

SCHILLER

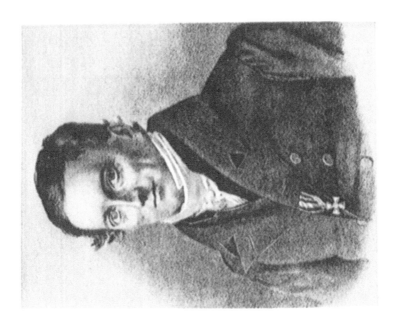

HERBART

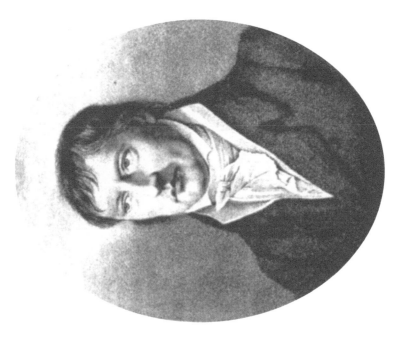

HEGEL

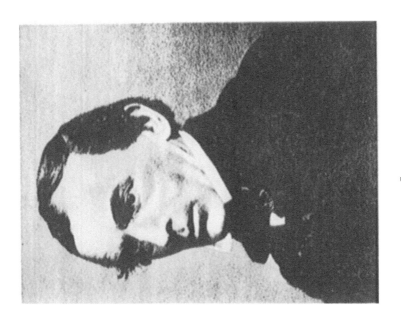

Lotze

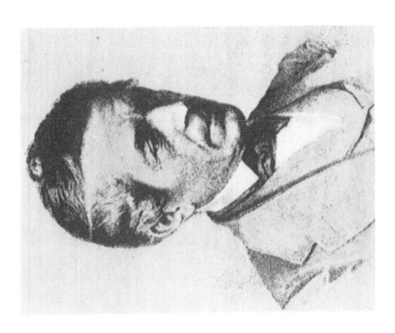

D. F. Strauss

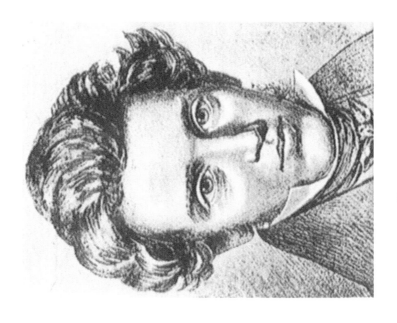

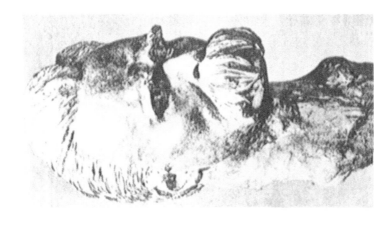

II. DOCTORS AND BIOLOGISTS

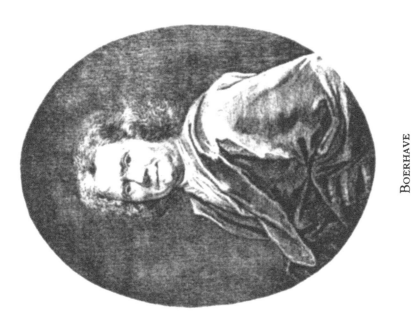

BOERHAVE

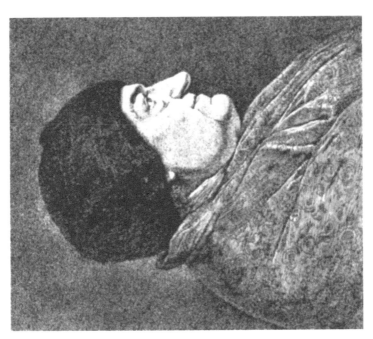

A. von HALLER

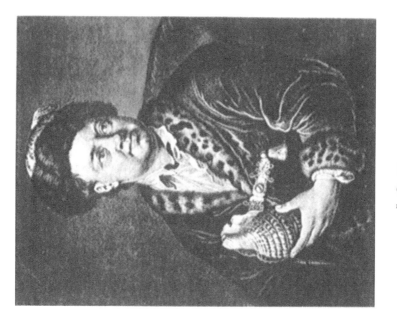

J. G. Gmelin

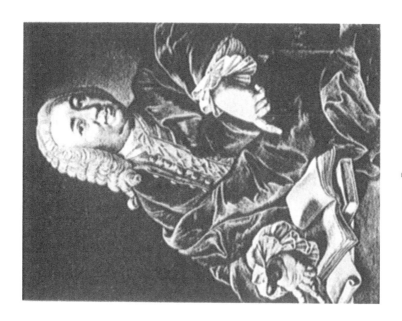

van Swieten

216

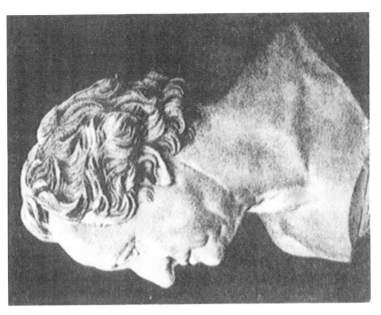

GOETHE

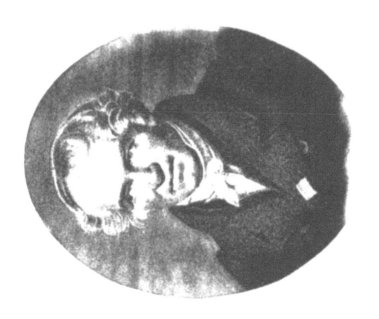

ALEXANDER VON HUMBOLDT

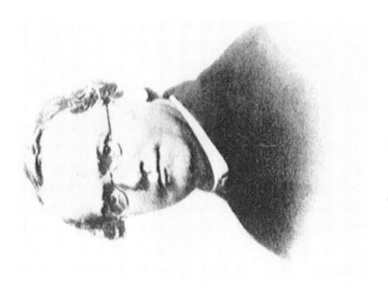

GREGOR MENDEL

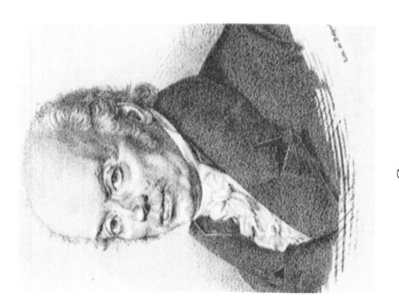

GALL

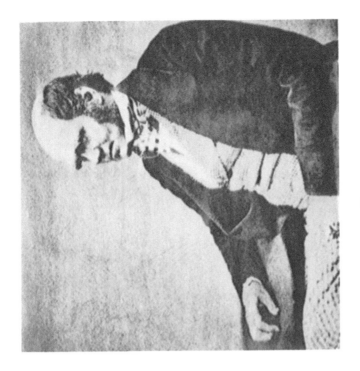

DARWIN

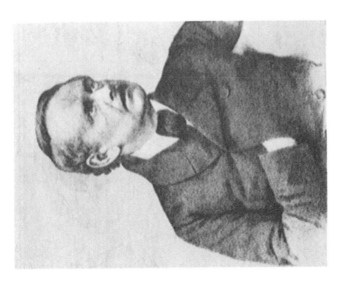

SCHLEIDEN

219

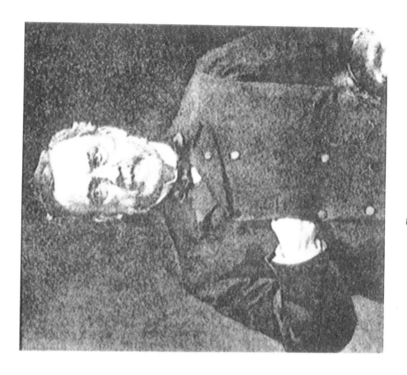

PASTEUR

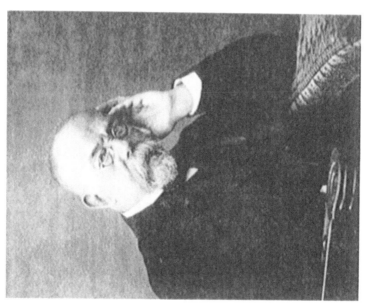

ROBERT KOCH

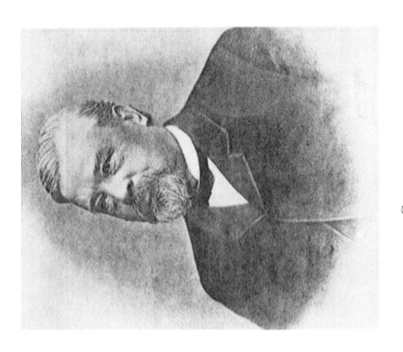

GEGENBAUR

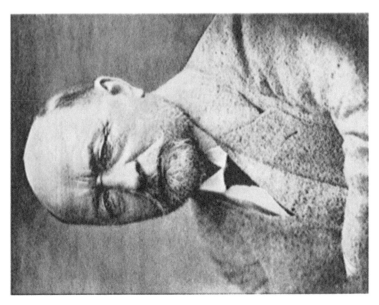

BEHRING

221

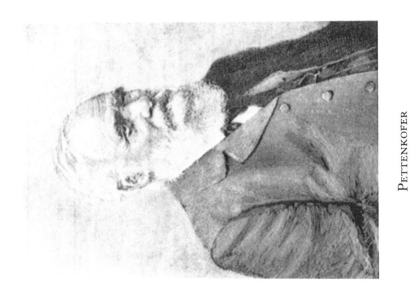

PETTENKOFER

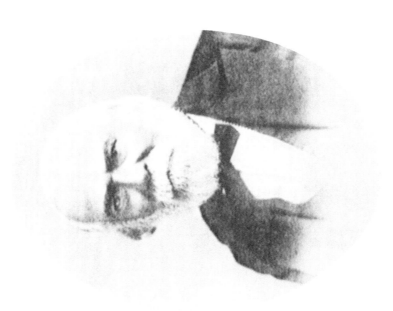

BROWN-SÉQUARD

222

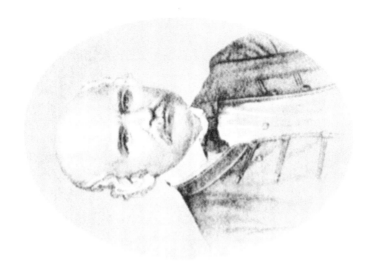

SEMMELWEIS

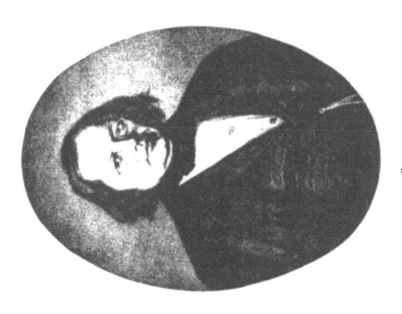

SKODA

223

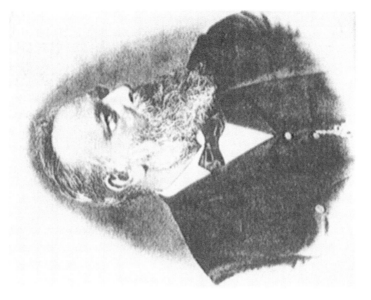

BILLROTH

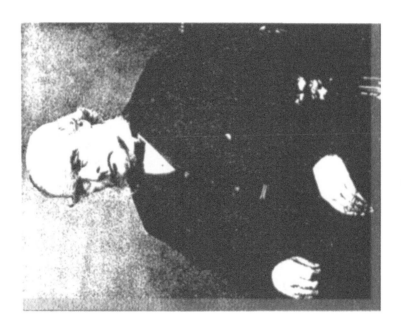

LISTER

224

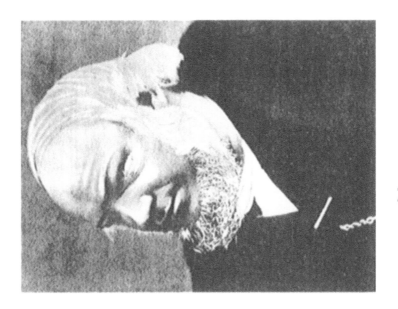

Moleschott

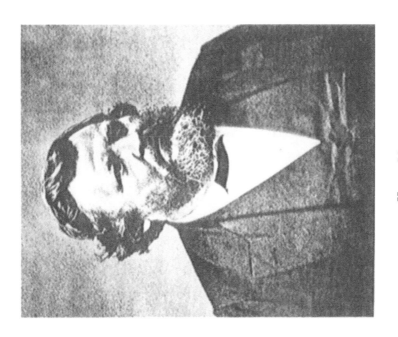

Karl Vogt

225

III. DRAMATISTS AND WRITERS OF TRAGEDY.

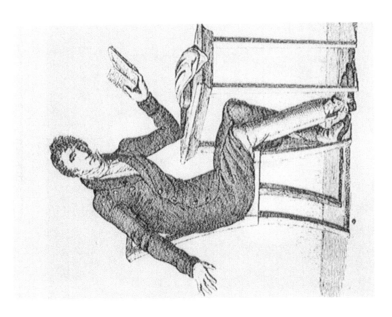

Zacharias Werner

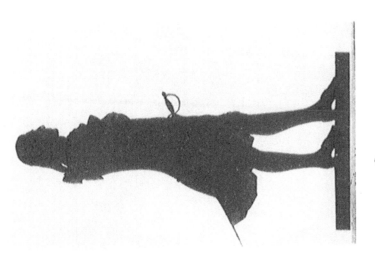

Schiller

229

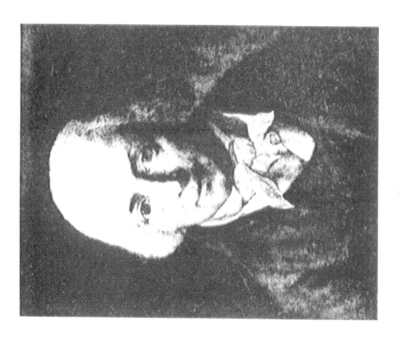

BÜRGER

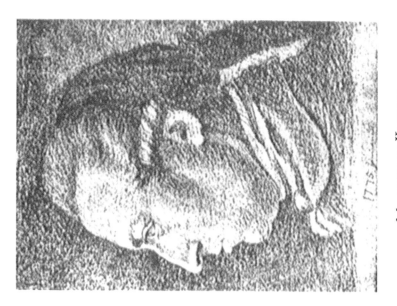

MAXIMILIAN KLINGER

230

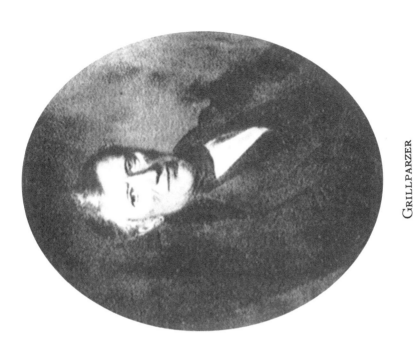

GRILLPARZER

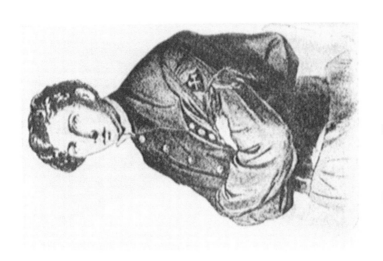

THEODOR KÖRNER

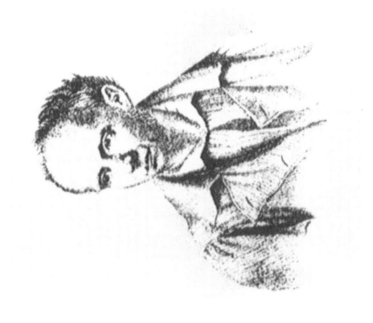

GRABBE

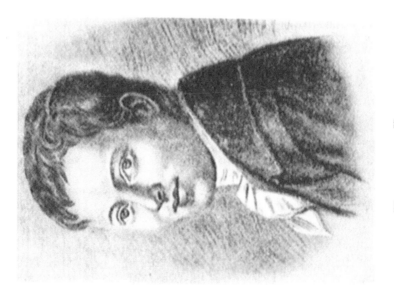

HEINRICH V. KLEIST

232

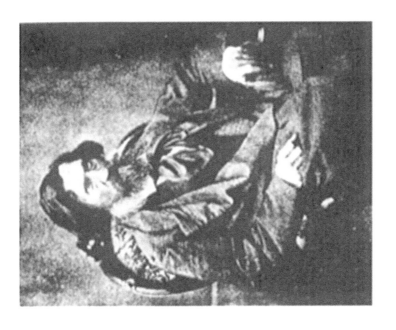

Otto Ludwig

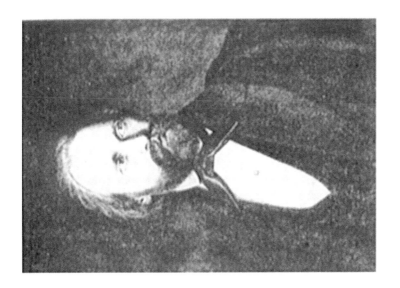

Friedrich Hebbel

233

IV. ROMANTICS AND STYLISTS

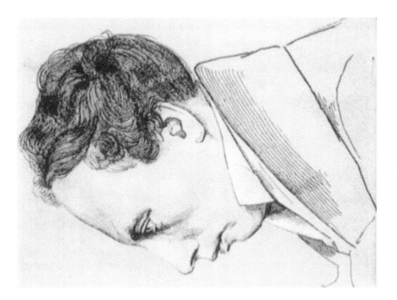

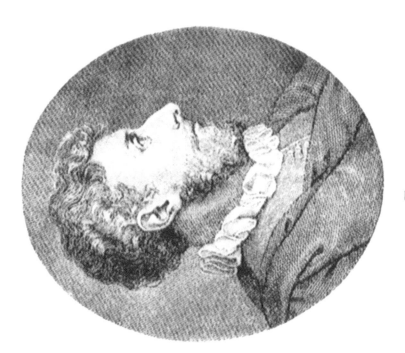

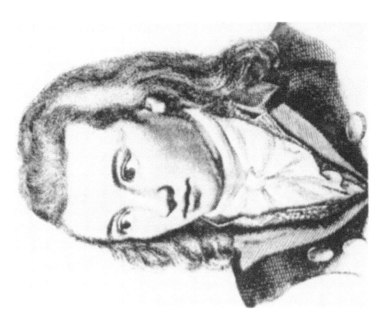

NOVALIS

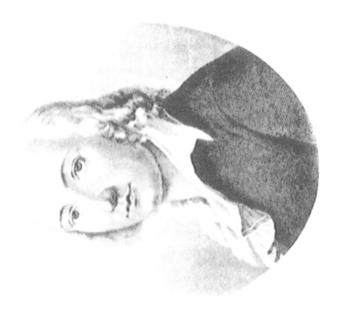

HÖLDERLIN

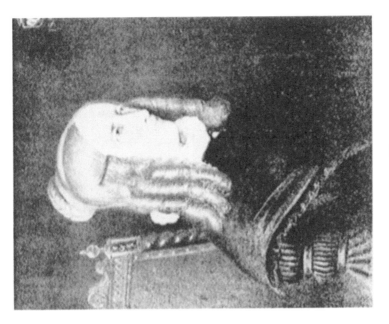

DROSTE-HÜLSHOFF

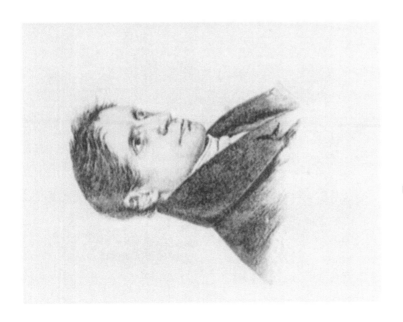

EICHENDORFF

239

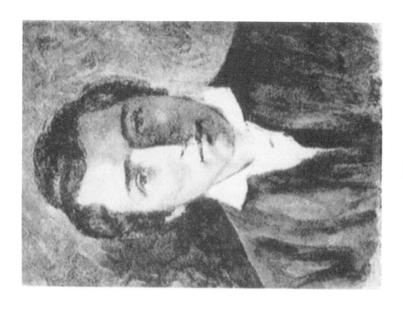

HEINE

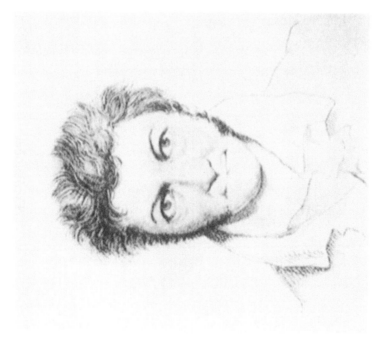

E. TH. A. HOFFMAN

240

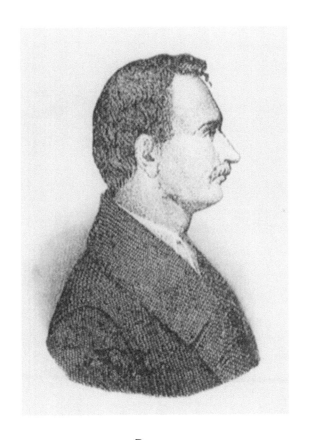

PLATEN

V. REALISTS AND HUMOURISTS

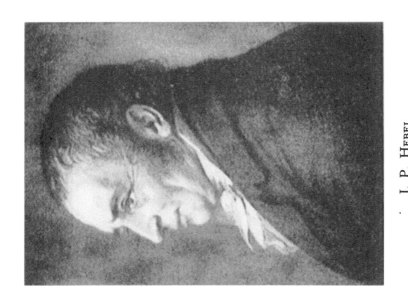

J. P. Hebel

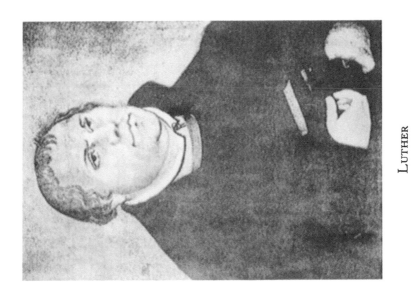

Luther

245

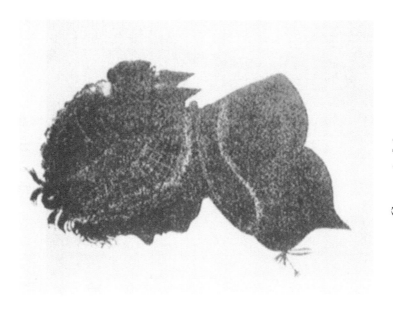

GOETHE's MOTHER.

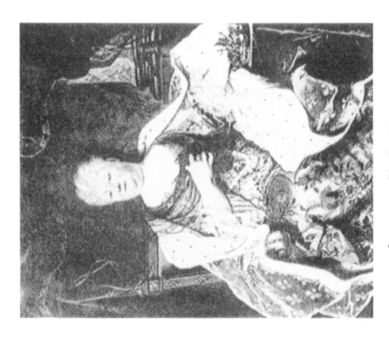

LISELOTTE V. D. PFALZ

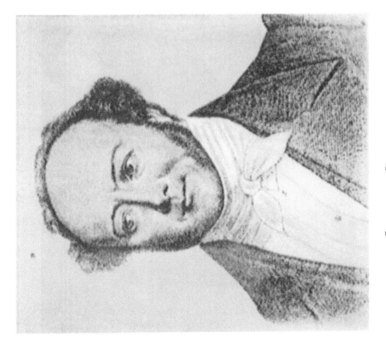

GOTTFRIED KELLER

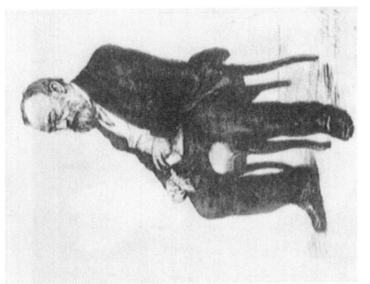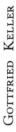

JEREMIAS GOTTHELF

247

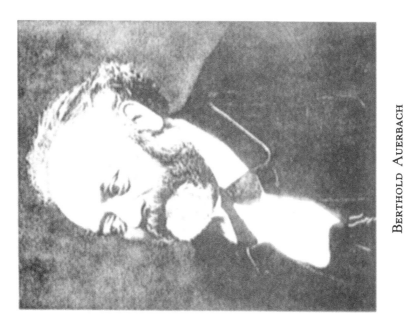

Berthold Auerbach

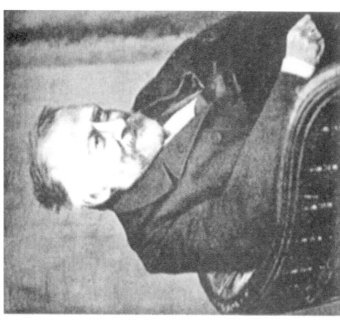

W. Alexis

248

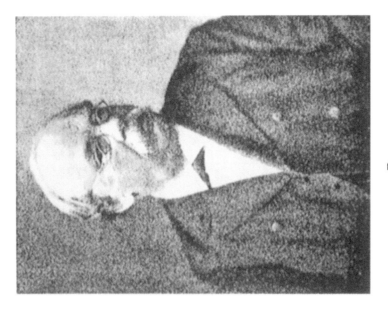

RIEHL

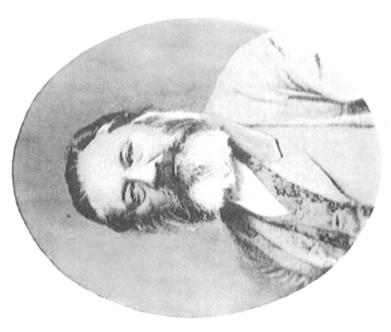

HERMANN KURZ

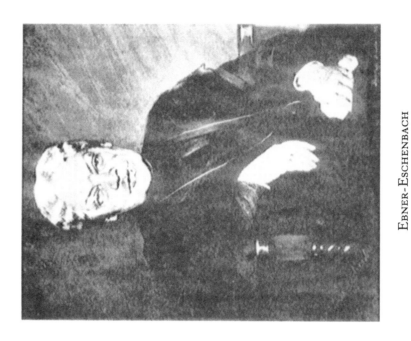

EBNER-ESCHENBACH

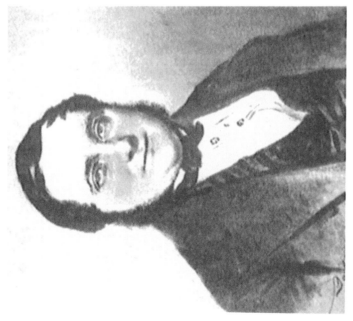

STIFTER

250

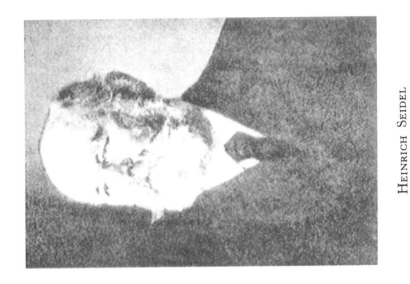

Heinrich Seidel

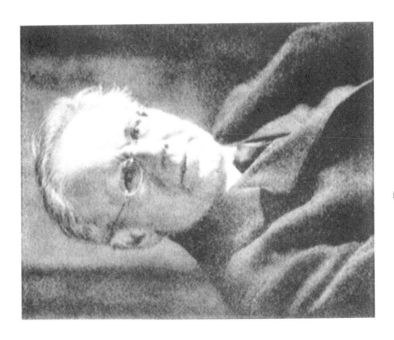

Rosegger

251

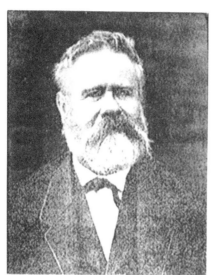
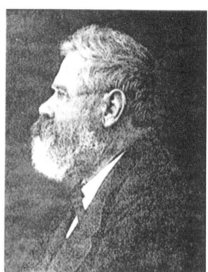

FRITZ REUTER

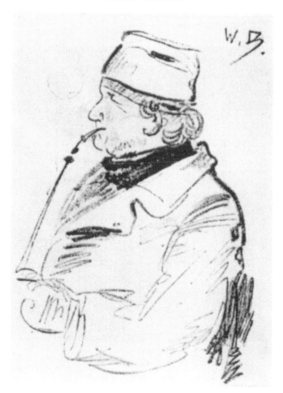

FATHER OF WILHELM BUSCH

SOURCES OF THE PORTRAIT COLLECTION

BIESE, Deutsche Literaturgeschichte. München: Beck.

BRUCKER-HAID, Bildersaal 1741.

Galerie hervorragender Ärzte und Naturforscher (Beilage zur Münch. Med. Wochenschr., München: Lehmann.)

LAVATER, Physiognomische Fragmente.

Minerva, biographisches Jahrbuch. Berlin: Reimer.

PAGEL, Biographisches Lexikon hervorragender Ärzte. Berlin: Urban und Schwarzenberg 1901.

VOGEL, J., Anton Graff. Leipzig: Breitkopf und Härtel 1898.

WERCKMEISTER, Das 19. Jahrhundert in Bildnissen. Berlin 1901.

WERKSHAGEN, Der Protestantismus.

The portraits reproduced in this book which are not to be found in the above mentioned works are taken from such sources as old prints, biographies, editions of the classics, etc.

INDEX